MY LIFE WITH

Healthcare series

MY LIFE WITH
DIABETES

Jan de Vries

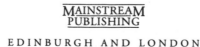
MAINSTREAM
PUBLISHING

EDINBURGH AND LONDON

First published in Great Britain in 2003 by
MAINSTREAM PUBLISHING (EDINBURGH) LTD
7 Albany Street
Edinburgh EH1 3UG

ISBN 1 84018 719 0

A catalogue record for this book is available from the British Library

Typeset in Baskerville MT

Printed in Great Britain by
Cox & Wyman Ltd

Contents

List of Tables

Foreword

Few people are famous and even fewer command respect, but how many are both adored and renowned worldwide? Jan de Vries is one of the members of that distinguished club. But what is his secret? Since his childhood, this world expert on alternative medicine has been tirelessly contributing to humanity through his vast knowledge, experience and, most of all, his compassion for those seeking a more holistic approach to managing both disease and wellness.

I count it both an honour and a privilege to have spent time with Jan discussing the promising research that will affect healthcare around the world in the years to come. We want what works best: prevention first, treatment that is effective and safe when needed, and the ability to choose therapies that complement each other and produce the best results.

In his latest book, he shares with us exciting new research, along with his own personal experience in managing diabetes. This is a 'must read' for everyone, as most of us know someone who is affected – read, learn and enjoy!

Abulkalam M. Shamsuddin, MD, PhD,
Professor of Pathology, University of Maryland
School of Medicine, USA

~ CHAPTER ONE ~

How Did I Get Diabetes?

In lectures, I often emphasise the point that we have three bodies, not one: a physical body, a mental body and an emotional body. If the three bodies are all working in harmony, very few health problems will arise. However, if just one is out of balance, they are all affected.

I have worked for over 18 years at 10 Harley Street in London and, as people from all over the world come to consult me there, it is an extremely busy clinic. On one occasion, after two hectic days of consulting at Harley Street, I flew to Australia straight from the clinic. That day had started off with the postman bringing me a letter from Canada that had greatly upset me, and that I realised later on had affected me emotionally. After my clinic, I rushed to Heathrow Airport to catch the plane to Sydney only to be told that I could not get a seat in the non-smoking area; unless I travelled first class, I would have no alternative but to sit in the smoking section. Travelling first class is against my principles, as I feel I am no better than anyone else, so I had to endure the smoky atmosphere on the plane for the entire flight, lasting 20 hours – that was the second attack on the three bodies that I am talking about, this time on my physical body. The lady who sat next to me on the plane chatted constantly and chain-smoked all the way from London to Sydney, the like of which I have never seen. In that sort of situation, I would normally have talked about the harmful effects of smoking, but as she was clearly nervous, I felt it would not have been fair to do so on that occasion. She was so stressed that, even in the middle of the flight, she asked if she could hold my hand as she was shaking. Although the smoke was unbearable, I had to be sensitive to her emotional needs.

When the three bodies are in balance, the immune system is strengthened. However, my immune system had already been attacked by a very busy day that had started with my receiving the upsetting letter, followed by the smoky atmosphere all the way to Sydney. Then, two hours after stepping off the plane, I gave a big lecture, which put strain on my mental body. A lot of things are bad for the body, so every aspect has to be examined carefully in order to look after our physical, mental and emotional selves so that a strong immunity can be created to maintain healthy living.

Anyway, the lecture in Sydney went well. The following day, I had promised to give a talk in the Australian bush about the characteristics and signatures of plants and flowers, and the roots and barks of trees. That, of course, was not easy, as I do not know a lot about plants and wildlife in the bush. I could only look at the characteristics and signatures of the plants and trees and, through my experience, explain how they developed and which medicinal values each one possessed. Not an easy task, especially with newspaper, radio and television reporters around me, all of whom asked some very awkward questions. I really had to make sure that I got my facts right.

I actually managed this very well and, after a few days, left the bush and travelled on to Melbourne to do a difficult lecture, attended by a lot of constitutional homoeopaths who asked some equally awkward questions. During it, I began to feel very unwell and started to shake. I managed to finish the talk and by the end, friends of mine luckily noticed I was not at all well and came on to the platform to help. I have known the actor Sir John

Mills and his wife very well for many years and during that time have also been friendly with his daughters, Hayley and Juliet Mills, who happened to be performing in Australia at that time and had fortunately known that I was giving this talk and come along. They felt something had to be done, as I looked so unwell, and indeed I ended up in an Australian hospital – the last place I wanted to be. The consultant was very friendly and, after some tests, came to the conclusion that while I was in the bush I must have picked up a virus from which I was not immune. To my great shock, he also told me that I had viral pneumonia and was very ill, so I should really stay in hospital. When he said that he needed to administer antibiotics I told him I was allergic to them and could not risk taking them. In that case, he then proceeded to tell me, I could not stay in the hospital, as he had seen me on television the previous day on my tour through the bush – because of my high profile he could not have me dying in an Australian hospital! He was very concerned, but I told him that I would go back to the hotel and take high doses of *Echinaforce*, originally formulated by Dr Alfred Vogel. I felt extremely ill by the time I arrived back in my room and must have taken almost a full bottle of *Echinaforce* during the night. I also administered all the forms of hydrotherapy with cold and hot water that I could. At five o'clock in the morning, believe it or not, the very nice consultant came to my room to see if I was still alive! He told me he had been very worried about me and could not sleep. He took great care of me, for which I shall always be grateful.

I cannot describe the kind of night I had, but I was certainly in a crisis and prayed hard to God not to let me die in Australia. All I wanted was to go back to my home in Scotland. However, when the consultant came to see me again later that day he was surprised at how quickly I was improving. I did my very best to get over that unpleasant experience, as I wanted to get back to work – I was only in Australia for three days. The consultant gave me a letter for my doctor in Scotland and made me promise him that when I returned, I would go to see the doctor. I was grateful that I recovered from that situation so fast and was soon well enough to finish my work in Australia.

I kept my promise to visit a doctor when I returned to Troon. As I had very seldom been before, I went to one I knew quite well. He took one look at me, then looked at the letter and said, 'You have to go to hospital. You need a thorough check-up.' I have always said that hospitals are good for diagnosing illnesses; they have all the equipment to hand, so that a thorough examination can be carried out to find the cause of the problem. I went to the hospital and had excellent care, and when I returned later to get the results, I was given the news that the glucose intolerance tests indicated my blood sugar was 33 – very high. In other words, I was diabetic. This was an enormous shock.

The sympathetic consultant I saw told me that if I did not adhere to strict orthodox treatment, it could be disastrous for me. I asked him nicely if he would allow me six weeks without medication to treat myself, as long as I monitored the situation, and he agreed. Within six weeks, I managed to get my blood sugar down to eight. He was very surprised at this, shook his head in disbelief and asked me what I had done. I asked him to give me some more time to see if things could be improved further, that he could not argue with my results, but that I would do as he asked if I could not control my condition with dietary management and some of my own remedies.

Now, I am not suggesting that diabetics should do without their pills or insulin injections in order to explore other avenues, as that would be very dangerous and should only be done if monitored by a doctor and a diabetes consultant. However, I have often seen that some diabetics who were insulin-dependent have been able to change to tablets through alternative methods of controlling the condition, and some have even managed to come off the tablets altogether. Following a strict dietary regime, which I will talk about in Chapter Six, is very important and will help diabetics feel much better.

So there I was, now knowing that I had diabetes and taking action to improve things. I learned a lot from that experience and realised that one cannot gamble with one's immune system – it is impossible. I learned that, as I had overdone things during that particular time in my life, my immune system couldn't fight off the unknown virus which I had contracted in the bush. Firstly there was my very busy lifestyle and my taxing days in Harley Street, then the letter that emotionally upset me and the physical attack of the smoky atmosphere in the plane, followed by a hectic programme of lecturing. I am sure that my immune system said, 'I have had enough – you must do it yourself.' From that moment on, and more and more over the years, I have realised how necessary it is to look after oneself. It is for that reason that I have written nearly 40 books during the 45 years I have been in practice. These books are based on results I have witnessed and how often I have seen people abuse themselves by neglecting their health, which can result in very serious problems. I had physically attacked myself by working too hard and then sitting in a smoky atmosphere, mentally overstretched myself and also put myself under a lot of emotional strain, which culminated in an imbalance. Building a good immune system depends greatly on being able to withstand attacks from the polluted air we breathe and the polluted foods we eat. It is quite surprising how wonderful the body is and how it can cope with these pollutants as long as we take care of our health and recognise that it is our own responsibility.

We can learn a little about the management of diabetes if we understand what diabetes really is. In the next chapter, I will talk about it and explain the condition. Later I will show what alternatives are available to us to help improve our diabetic condition and maintain good health. None of the doctors or dieticians can believe that, by taking my own prescribed medicines and by dietary management, my blood sugar could be reduced from 33 to now roughly 7 or, at the highest, 8. I have maintained this level for quite a number of years and to the surprise of many, can still work over 90 hours a week. It really doesn't take a lot of effort to keep my diabetes under control.

~ CHAPTER TWO ~

What is Diabetes?

Some time ago I was waiting for a delayed flight to take off from Stansted Airport. There were intermittent messages, first of all relaying various reasons for the problem and explaining what was wrong with the plane, then saying that there would be a one-hour delay, then almost two hours, then that there was congestion of air traffic. This, added to the heavy schedule I had in front of me, made it easy to see how one could get frustrated. Frustration is one of the worst emotions for diabetics, as it can cause the blood sugar to rise.

Near me in the airport, also waiting for the flight, I saw a very charming, pretty lady whose face was getting more and more red with each frustrating message. I couldn't help saying to her that there was nothing either of us could do – we just had to learn to accept that travelling is not as it used to be. We started to talk and she told me that she spent a lot of time travelling and that this sort of experience was not good for her, as she was diabetic. I had found a fellow sufferer who understood. I could see that she was a very intelligent lady who I imagined was very good at her work, so I was surprised when she asked me the simple question, 'What is diabetes really?' There was a lot of time to wait for the plane so we talked about our mutual problem then and later too, during the flight. In very simple terms, I explained to her a little bit about what diabetes really is. She was most interested.

Like myself, her main problem was regulating the blood sugar, which often fluctuated; she had difficulty balancing it. When I looked at her and carried out a Chinese facial diagnosis, I could see that she had a thyroid problem and asked her if she had trouble with her weight. Indeed, I was correct – that was one of her main problems. Often with diabetic patients, the weight fluctuates, especially at a higher level, but it is very important to keep it down as the blood sugar is very dependent on it. This was one of the lady's biggest problems and I asked her if I could take her on as a case study. I found it very interesting to see that it was not only the pancreas that is implicated in diabetes (as was the case with myself during my experience in Australia, when I was told that my pancreas had been damaged by the viral attack), but that every endocrine gland is affected when one of them is out of harmony. In this lady, the imbalance was very much implicated in her weight problem.

We had an interesting conversation and I told her a little bit about the pancreas which, next to the liver, is the most important organ in the digestive system. Although the pancreas is only one-twentieth of the size of the liver, it plays a very important role, where it touches the spleen and the left kidney. The secretion from the pancreas and salivary glands is very concentrated and the digestive enzymes in this fluid have a vital function. When the stomach fills, the pancreas has an effect on the stomach's workload. This is one of the reasons that it is very important to keep the weight down – the more overweight you are, the harder your pancreas has to work. The enzyme diastase, or amylase, changes starch into sugars, such as glycogen, dextrin and maltose. Trypsin, like pepsin, breaks down the proteins into peptones and, finally, into the basic building blocks of proteins and amino acids. The fourth enzyme, lipase, together with the bowel, hydrolyses fats into fatty acids and glycerol. In fact, the body cannot break down, digest and assimilate protein, starches and fats without the enzymes secreted by the pancreas. Alfred Vogel, in his book *The Nature Doctor*, says that 'neither the bowel nor the pancreatic enzymes are fully efficient if the juice in the small intestine and the bacterial flora are not normal'. It is sometimes very difficult to understand these facts, but it is important to know about the wonderful interplay of digestive organs in the glandular system. Harmony is very important in this system and the relationships are fully automatic. When we eat, it is quite amazing how a message is sent via the nerves to the cerebellum, and instantaneously another message is sent to the intestines, the liver and the pancreas. Enzymes from the pancreas are immediately needed in this process.

The embedded cell formations in the pancreas are shaped like blackberries. They are small glands, but not at all connected with other glands. Like islets in the bigger gland, they are called the islets of Langerhans, after Paul Langerhans, who discovered them. The vital substance, insulin, is produced in these small glands and sent straight into the bloodstream, not to the small intestines. If these islets do not manufacture sufficient insulin, glycogen (the sugar stored in the liver and passed to the blood in accordance with the body's needs) will not be utilised, so that the blood sugar level rises. The excess is excreted through the kidneys, which is why sugar is found in the urine. This is a symptom of the disease known as diabetes.

As I told my fellow passenger, that is basically what diabetes is. Later on in this chapter, I will explain it in more depth. It is most important that one takes proper care of the pancreas and I learned only too well how very careful one has to be with this marvellous gland which is so small, but so vital. The lady in question was very diet-conscious and I was impressed by how well informed she was on dietary management. Not only that, she was very disciplined in her eating habits. She told me that she and her husband often had to attend social functions because of their jobs, but that she was always vigilant about her diet. This is, of course, very important, especially for her, since I had noticed that the thyroid was a contributory factor. I will explain later how the thyroid works in harmony with the rest of the endocrine glands. A lot of diabetic patients have digestive problems and need help to make the pancreas function efficiently.

This lady agreed to my taking her on as a case study and she followed my advice to the letter. I saw immediately that she responded to the excellent remedy *Molkosan*, one of the supplements that it is extremely necessary for a diabetic to take. Its main ingredient is whey, the only milk product I really like for health reasons. It is the leftover from cheese-making, and is not only a great antiseptic but also helps the pancreas produce more natural insulin. It benefited this particular lady tremendously and also helped her to control her weight. I also gave her several other remedies, such as *Doctor's Choice for Diabetics*, which is a brilliant American product, and *Diabetisan*, another remedy from Alfred Vogel, both of which are helpful. So too are salads made with *Molkosan*, blueberry juice and blackcurrant juice as a dressing. Breathing exercises for relaxation and a few other remedies to control this lady's weight were also extremely beneficial. She made a remarkable recovery and her blood sugar became much more balanced. Although she was not terribly overweight, it was still difficult to deal with because of the influence of the thyroid. We still concentrate on this in her treatment, but she has so much more vitality and energy now as a result of following some of the methods I shall discuss in this book, and those she followed to the letter.

Even though it was difficult, she realised that fasting was an excellent means of resting the pancreas. It is important that one should eat small quantities and chew everything thoroughly, so that the saliva can mix with food, as saliva is still the best digestive material. It is very important to eat carefully and fasting works very well along with regular deep-breathing exercises.

Many serious problems can be prevented if the proper function of the pancreas is restored, and a diabetic can lead a much easier life. I still see this lady regularly and will keep working with her until we have achieved harmony between all seven endocrine glands. In her case, the pancreas was her greatest problem and the influence on the thyroid gland was another. It even showed in her eyes; we can see by using iridology how the endocrine glands work. There are seven endocrine glands, there are seven light receptors in the eye, seven colours in the rainbow and seven basic scale steps in a musical octave. These have to work in harmony, and not only do I have to take care of this lady's pancreas, but also of her thyroid because, in her case, the thyroid had prevented the hormonal balance. The thyroid is like a gatekeeper. If its hormones function at sub-optimal levels, nothing else in the body tends to work well either. Low thyroid function (hypothyroidism) leaves the body vulnerable to allergies, autoimmune disorders, cancer, chronic fatigue, diabetes, elevated cholesterol, emotional behaviour problems, emphysema, high blood pressure, hypoglycaemia, infectious diseases, menstrual disorders, migraine headaches, premature ageing and skin conditions. Low thyroid function may be one of the most undiagnosed of all conditions. Laboratory tests for measuring it are unreliable, because they reveal if the thyroid gland is diseased but not if the thyroid hormones are functioning at sub-optimal levels. Thyroid hormones circulating in the bloodstream do not necessarily reach all the cells that need them. Thyroxine (T4), the active hormone in the thyroid gland, is made from iodine and amino acids. Nutrients that contribute to the manufacture and release of thyroid hormones include vitamin E. Taking supplementary amounts of vitamin E can help to restore normal thyroid function.

These were a few of the things that had to be taken into account when I was treating this lovely lady, who works almost as hard as I do. She is always so grateful for the way she has been helped to cope with her diabetes and the amount of energy she now has.

Now we come to the big question – what *is* diabetes? To explain this further, we will look at a few questions and answers.

Diabetes is a chronic disorder of carbohydrate, fat and protein metabolism characterised by increased levels of blood sugar (glucose) and a greatly increased risk of heart disease, stroke, kidney disease and loss of nerve function. Diabetes can occur when the pancreas does not secrete enough insulin, or if the cells of the body become resistant to insulin; the blood sugar cannot reach the cells, leading to serious complications.

Diabetes is divided into two major categories: Type I and Type II. Type I, or Insulin-Dependent Diabetes Mellitus (IDDM), occurs most often in children and adolescents. Type II or Non Insulin-Dependent Diabetes Mellitus (NIDDM) occurs most frequently in adults over 40 years of age.

HOW COMMON IS DIABETES?

Using the United States as an example, the overall frequency rate of diabetes is estimated at approximately 4.5 per cent, of which 90 per cent are Type II and the rest Type I. In 1992, while diabetics accounted for only 4.5 per cent of the US population, their care required roughly 14.6 per cent of the total US healthcare expenditure ($105 billion). The number of Americans with diabetes is rising. It is now the seventh leading cause of death in the US. At the current rate of increase (6 per cent per year), the number of diabetics will double every 15 years. Population studies have linked diabetes to diet and lifestyle. Diabetes is uncommon in cultures consuming a more 'primitive' diet. As cultures switch from their native diets to the highly processed 'foods of commerce', their rate of diabetes increases, eventually reaching the proportion seen in Western societies.

WHAT ARE THE SYMPTOMS OF DIABETES?

The classic symptoms of diabetes are frequent urination and excessive thirst and appetite. Because these symptoms are not very serious, many people with diabetes do not seek medical care. In fact, it is thought that fewer than half of all diabetic Americans (estimated at more than 10 million) know that they have the condition or ever consult a doctor.

WHAT CAUSES DIABETES?

Type I diabetes is associated with the complete destruction of the beta cells, which manufacture the hormone insulin, in the pancreas. Type I patients require lifelong insulin for the control of blood sugar levels. The Type I diabetic must learn how to manage his or her blood sugar levels on a day-to-day basis, modifying insulin types and dosage schedules as necessary, according to the results of regular blood sugar testing. About 10 per cent of all diabetics are Type I. Although the exact cause of Type I diabetes is unknown, current theory suggests it is caused by injury to the insulin-producing beta cells that results when the body's immune system begins attacking the pancreas. Antibodies for beta cells are present in 75 per cent of all cases of Type I diabetes compared to the normal 0.5 per cent to 2.0 per cent. It is probable that the antibodies to the beta cells develop in response to cell destruction due to other mechanisms (chemical, free radical, viral, food allergy, etc.). It appears that normal individuals either do not develop as severe an antibody reaction, or are better able to repair the damage once it occurs.

In Type II diabetes, insulin levels are typically elevated, indicating a loss of sensitivity to insulin by the cells of the body. Obesity is a major contributing factor to this loss of insulin sensitivity, with approximately 90 per cent of individuals with Type II diabetes being obese. When a good body weight is achieved by Type II patients, normal blood sugar levels are usually restored. In the treatment of Type II diabetes, diet is of primary importance and should be diligently followed before a drug is used. Most Type II diabetes can be controlled by diet alone. Despite a high success rate with dietary intervention, doctors often use drugs or insulin instead.

Table 1: Comparison of Type I and Type II Diabetes

Features	Type I	Type II
Age at onset	Usually under 40	Usually over 40

per cent of all diabetics	Fewer than 10 per cent	Greater than 90 per cent
Seasonal trend	Autumn and winter	None
Family history	Uncommon	Common
Appearance of symptoms	Rapid	Slow
Obesity at onset	Uncommon	Common
Insulin levels	Decreased	Variable
Insulin resistance	Occasional	Often
Treatment with insulin	Always	Not required
Beta cells	Decreased	Variable
Ketoacidosis	Frequent	Rare
Complications	Frequent	Frequent

WHY IS IT IMPORTANT TO MONITOR BLOOD SUGAR LEVELS?

The likelihood of developing complications, whether acute or chronic, is ultimately a reflection of the level of blood sugar control. A large body of evidence indicates that good blood sugar control significantly reduces the development of complications. Therefore, monitoring and controlling blood sugar levels is critical to the prevention of the major diabetic complications.

WHAT ARE THE MAJOR COMPLICATIONS OF DIABETES?

Although the acute complications, such as ketoacidosis (a state of absolute insulin deprivation), are more serious in the short term, the long-term consequences of diabetes are just as deadly. The major long-term complications of diabetes are atherosclerosis (hardening of the arteries), diabetic retinopathy (eye disease), diabetic neuropathy (nerve damage), diabetic nephropathy (kidney disease) and diabetic foot ulcers.

WHAT NUTRITIONAL SUPPLEMENTS ARE IMPORTANT TO DIABETICS?

The diabetic has an increased need for many nutrients and

several have also been shown to be important in preventing some of the long-term complications of diabetes. For example, since vitamin C requires insulin for transport into cells, most diabetics suffer from impaired vitamin C metabolism and diabetics with neuropathy have been shown to be deficient in vitamin B6 and to benefit from supplementation. Individuals with longstanding diabetes or who are developing signs of peripheral nerve abnormalities should definitely be supplemented with vitamins C and B6, and other key nutrients. Table 2 lists some of the key nutrients.

Table 2: Key Nutrients for Diabetics

Chromium	Low levels may lead to insulin insensitivity
Vitamins C and E	Increased requirements
Magnesium	Increased requirements, improves all aspects
Biotin	Activates glucokinase, promotes glucose utilisation
Vitamin B6	Prevents and improves neuropathy
Methylcobalamin (B12)	Prevents and improves neuropathy
Zinc, manganese, vanadyl	Improves insulin action
Gamma-linolenic acid	Prevents and improves neuropathy
Pantethine	Improves cell membrane and blood lipid levels

ARE THERE ANY NUTRIENTS THAT CAN HELP REVERSE IDDM?

Supplementing the diet of recently diagnosed Type I diabetics with niacin in the form of niacinamide (also called nicotinamide) has been shown to prevent the development of IDDM as well as lead to reversal in some cases. There have been ten studies of niacinamide treatment in recent-onset Type I diabetes, or Type I of less than five years' duration. Six of these studies used a double-blind, placebo-controlled format. Of these six, three studies showed a positive effect in terms of prolonged remission, lower insulin requirements, improved metabolic control and increased beta cell function. Some newly diagnosed Type I diabetics have experienced complete reversal of their diabetes with niacinamide supplementation. In the spring of 1993, a large multi-centre study involving 18 European countries, Israel and Canada was started to follow up these encouraging preliminary findings. Other clinical trials are also in progress or have been proposed. The mechanism of action appears to be inhibition of damage to the insulin-producing cells by the immune system along with niacinamide's antioxidant role. The daily dose of niacinamide is based on body weight, 25 mg per kilogram. The studies in children used 100 mg to 200 mg per day. It is certainly worth a try.

WHAT ROLE DOES CHROMIUM PLAY IN DIABETES?

The trace mineral chromium plays a major role in the sensitivity of cells to insulin. Chromium, as a critical component of the so-called 'glucose tolerance factor' (GTF), functions as a co-factor in all insulin-regulating activities. Chromium deficiency is widespread in the United States. Supplementing the diet with chromium has been shown to significantly improve insulin action, decrease glucose, cholesterol and triglyceride levels, and increase the HDL-cholesterol level by increasing insulin sensitivity in normal, elderly and Type II patients. Chromium is not, however, a cure-all for Type II diabetes. In other words, although chromium is important and many cases of Type II diabetes will be improved by chromium supplementation, it will only produce its benefits in people with low chromium levels. Clinical studies in diabetics have shown that supplementing the diet with chromium decreases glucose levels, improves glucose tolerance, lowers insulin levels and decreases total cholesterol and triglyceride levels, while increasing HDL-cholesterol levels. Although some studies have not shown chromium to exert much effect in improving glucose tolerance in diabetics, there is no doubt that it is an important mineral in blood sugar metabolism.

ARE HERBAL MEDICINES HELPFUL IN DIABETES?

Yes. Before the advent of insulin, diabetes was treated with plant medicines. In 1980, the World Health Organisation urged researchers to examine whether traditional medicines produced any beneficial clinical results. In the last 10 to 20 years, scientific investigation has, in fact, confirmed the benefits of many of these preparations. I would recommend that diabetics utilise a high-quality garlic preparation, a comprehensive multi-vitamin and mineral formula, bitter melon extract, gymnema sylvestre extract and either bilberry, grape seed or ginkgo extract. By a high-quality garlic preparation, I mean one that is standardised to deliver an allicin content of at least 4,000 mcg per day.

WARNING: Under no circumstances should a person stop taking diabetic drugs, especially insulin, unless he or she is being closely monitored by a doctor.

WHAT ABOUT DIET AND EXERCISE?

Dietary modification and treatment is fundamental to the successful treatment of diabetes, whether it be Type I or II. The frequency of diabetes is highly correlated with the fibre-depleted, highly refined, high-carbohydrate diet of 'civilised' society. The most important dietary recommendation is to eliminate all sources of refined sugar and substitute these high-sugar foods with high-fibre, nutrient-rich foods. Especially beneficial are vegetables and legumes. As far as exercise goes, it is absolutely essential. Diabetics who exercise regularly experience many benefits: enhanced insulin sensitivity with a consequent diminished need for exogenous insulin, improved glucose tolerance, reduced total serum cholesterol and triglycerides and, in obese diabetics, improved weight loss.

WILL INSULIN OR DRUG DOSAGES CHANGE BY FOLLOWING YOUR SUPPLEMENT PROGRAMME?

Yes. I encourage you to develop a good working relationship with your doctor and strongly encourage you to monitor blood sugar levels carefully, particularly if you are on insulin or have poorly controlled diabetes. Home glucose monitoring and the glycosylated haemoglobin test are the best ways to monitor progress. It is important to recognise that as natural therapies take effect, insulin requirements and drug dosages will have to be altered.

A lot of time can be spent on explaining what diabetes really is. It is very important to learn to understand this disease and the need to manage it intelligently. A lot of research work has been done and the new information that results from this work always surprises me. Not long ago, researchers from the University of Pittsburgh, the graduate school of public health, discovered that women with long-term diabetes are at greater risk of premature menopause. The doctor who led the study said that the take-home message of the study for women with diabetes is that they should be extra vigilant about adopting a healthy heart and bone lifestyle by not smoking, exercising regularly, trying to maintain an ideal weight and keeping their diabetes under control. This is very good advice. Both men and women who are afflicted with this disease should take essential advice from their diabetes consultants, their general practitioners, dieticians and other experts who specialise in this disease, which is spreading very quickly.

~ CHAPTER THREE ~

What are the Alternatives?

When I left hospital with the knowledge that my blood sugar was 33 and pleaded with the consultant to give me time to bring it down using my own methods, I kept thinking of the promise I had made to him that if after six weeks I hadn't managed to get my blood sugar level reduced to his satisfaction, I would take the tablets that he advised, or even injections, and would do exactly as he instructed. I left him with the promise that I would do my very best and that if I felt unwell I would phone him, and he was most cooperative. He did say, however, that he would allow me six weeks only and then he would review the situation.

I took very swift action. I looked carefully at my diet and immediately cut out all sugar, bread and potatoes – this was drastic action, but I felt I had to do it. I then looked at the alternative remedies I could use to bring my blood sugar down quickly. I took *Doctor's Choice for Diabetics*, an American product which I knew was very helpful, together with Alfred Vogel's famous remedy *Diabetisan* (a herbal extract), *chromium* and *Molkosan*. These were the four things that I took and within a week I felt better. When I returned to the hospital to see the consultant, he was surprised to see that my blood sugar had reduced to around ten. However, he still wasn't happy, and said that if I took the pills, I would soon have it down to six or seven. I asked him if he would give me another six weeks to try and do so on my own and he agreed. After this further time had elapsed, I had managed to get it down to between seven and eight. Since then, I have been able to control my blood sugar levels by this method extremely well. I do not want my readers who are insulin dependent or on tablets to think that I am advising them to stop their current treatment and try my method, but what I will advise is that if you do decide to try this method, at first combined with your medication, you will soon see how much more stable your blood sugar will become. You can then discuss with your doctor or consultant how you can come off your medication. In the years that I have used alternative methods of controlling diabetes, I have seen some insulin-dependent patients go on to tablets and finally even come off the tablets and simply control things using alternative methods. Dietary management is terribly important and in Chapter Six I point out the great importance of diet – even to the extent that allowing a digestive biscuit can be disastrous. Therefore, I am always happy that the dieticians who control a diabetic's diet are well informed and can offer dietary advice, especially on the balance between carbohydrates and proteins. It is quite interesting that every person on earth is different and that an individual diet is very often the answer to controlling blood sugar.

So what are the alternatives? If we look into this, we can see that a tremendous choice is available, but particular attention should be paid to the products that have been established for the longest time. However, in saying that, I have recently been very encouraged by the findings of Prof. Shamsuddin that *inositol (IP-6)* has given the most remarkable results, and not only is this a great breakthrough for cancer patients, but it will also help diabetics. Prof. Shamsuddin is correct when he writes that cancer is a metabolic disease, but so is diabetes. It is interesting to note that this great man made this remarkable discovery from a simple food product, rice.

I will look at *inositol* in detail later in this chapter, but first of all, we will take a closer look at one product that I dearly love, the only milk product that I really like for health reasons, *Molkosan*. This remedy, which I have worked with now for almost 45 years, has often surprised me. It is made from the byproducts of cheese production. The whey of the milk is not only a great antiseptic, but also helps diabetics tremendously in assisting with the creation of more natural insulin. *Molkosan* is concentrated milk whey that not only maintains a healthy intestinal flora, but is also wonderful for diabetics. The yeast *candida albicans* is present in every individual. It normally lives harmlessly in the gastrointestinal tract. Antibiotics are often responsible for upsetting the balance of the intestinal flora by suppressing the normal intestinal bacteria. This provides an opportunity for candida overgrowth. The antifungal activity of *Molkosan* is due to its acidity and buffering capability. It is able to re-establish the normal balance of organisms in the digestive tract. This antifungal activity is also useful topically against vaginal thrush, athlete's foot and ringworm. The ability of orotic acid to enhance the digestive and metabolic processes makes *Molkosan* useful as an aid to a slimming programme.

The name *Molkosan* is derived from the German word for whey. It is a naturally lactofermented whey which is concentrated during processing to ensure a high content of minerals, especially calcium, potassium, phosphorus and L(+) lactic acid. L(+) lactic acid gives the product a pH of 2.7 (very acidic) which combines with its antiseptic action to inhibit bacterial and fungal infections. The lactose in *Molkosan* is present in its natural form, which does not cause digestive problems for lactose-intolerant or lactose-sensitive people.

The low acidity created by *Molkosan* promotes the growth of normal digestive tract flora. It also normalises intestinal flora that has been disturbed. *Molkosan* has been found to have anti-fungal activity. It can be applied directly to areas affected by fungal infections, such as athlete's foot, ringworm and thrush. Solutions of *Molkosan* in water are also effective against a variety of scalp complaints such as dandruff. It contains orotic acid, which is essential for the formation of DNA and RNA – the protein 'building block' of the body. Orotic acid combines with minerals to form orotates, which are easily absorbed by the body, acting as chemical buffers. These compounds help to create a beneficial environment, which is important to health. It is especially useful in a slimming programme, as fat metabolism creates breakdown products that need to be buffered or neutralised. As a slimming aid, *Molkosan* should be diluted: 15 ml to 100 ml of mineral water or diluted vegetable juice for maximum benefit.

For internal use: one teaspoon to a glass of mineral water, taken internally three times a day before or with meals.

For external use: apply to small wounds, abrasions and skin rashes, diluted to a ratio of 1:4 with water.

For insect bites: apply undiluted on the bite.

As a hair and body rinse: dilute *Molkosan* 1:10 with water and use this mixture to rinse hair and skin after showers. Do not rinse again with fresh water.

Duration of administration: there are no restrictions on the long-term use of this product and no known side effects. However, if you are pregnant or a nursing mother, *Molkosan* is not recommended unless directed by a healthcare professional.

Ingredients: fermented and concentrated milk whey.

Table 3: Nutrients in Molkosan

Total lactic acid	8,500 mg
L(+) lactic acid	7,000 mg
Lactose	4,000 mg
Total minerals	1,000 mg
Calcium	130 mg
Potassium	190 mg
Phosphorus	100 mg
Magnesium	trace
Zinc	trace

Iron	trace
Chloride	trace
Orotic acid	trace
Vitamin B complex	trace
Vitamin C	trace

Diabetisan is another fantastic remedy, concocted from several herbs by Alfred Vogel, and also has no known side effects. It was a tremendous help to me, taken twice a day, 15 drops, together with *chromium*. It contains:

Table 4: Nutrients in Diabetisan

Vaccinium myrtillus (bilberry)	22 per cent
Phaseolus nanus (kidney bean)	22 per cent
Medicago sativa (alfalfa)	22 per cent
Juglans regia (English walnut)	12 per cent
Potentilla erecta (tormentil)	11 per cent
Cardamine pratensis (cuckoo flower)	11 per cent
Alcohol content	52 per cent

Chromium picolinate is a trace mineral that plays an important part in the 'glucose tolerance factor', a critical enzyme system involved in blood sugar metabolism. Considerable evidence indicates that chromium levels help determine insulin sensitivity. Insulin helps cells to absorb and use glucose effectively. It may be useful in the treatment of impaired glucose tolerance, elevated blood cholesterol and triglyceride levels, promotion of weight loss, acne and PMS.

Each tablet contains 200 mcg of *chromium picolinate*. Other ingredients are cellulose, gelatin, magnesium stearate, silicon dioxide and titanium dioxide. It contains no sugar, salt, yeast, wheat, gluten, corn, soy, dairy products, colouring, flavouring or preservatives.

One capsule taken up to three times daily with food is the recommended dose and no side effects are known.

I have found this particular chromium supplement a terrific help in stabilising the blood sugar.

Possibly one of the best remedies available for diabetics is *Doctor's Choice for Diabetics*. Formulated by Enzymatic Therapy, it helps support the metabolic demands of a diabetic's system and is designed to ensure that all the special daily nutritional needs of a diabetic are met. This may help prevent some of the common health complications associated with a chronically elevated blood sugar level. For many diabetics, it is the distressing side effects of the condition, such as circulatory disturbance, premature heart disease, nerve damage (diabetic neuropathy) and sight degeneration that present most health problems. Modern nutritional research is now showing that attention to diet is a key aspect of managing diabetes, along with supplementation of specific nutrients and trace elements such as vanadium. The nutrients contained within *Doctor's Choice for Diabetics* include:

Vitamin E: supports connective tissue health and suppresses damaging free radicals associated with premature tissue degeneration.

Vitamin C: promotes healthy circulation and keeps blood 'thin'. May help slow the development of peripheral nerve complications and degeneration of the retina.

Vitamin B6: helps to keep fasting blood sugars level and may help prevent the onset of diabetic neuropathy.

Folic Acid: a key nutrient to help prevent premature heart disease by keeping levels of homocysteine – a known promoter of atherosclerosis and heart disease – down.

Vitamin B12: an important nutrient required for optimal nerve health.

Biotin: helps maintain a healthy skin as well as playing a controlling role in fat (lipogenesis) and glucose (gluconeogenesis) metabolism.

Zinc: important in the wound-healing process and helps speed recovery from illness.

Selenium: a key antioxidant mineral, works closely with vitamins C and E.

Chromium: one of the most important nutrients for a diabetic. Also known as the glucose tolerance factor, it greatly improves blood glucose fluctuations.

Gymnema sylvestre: a botanical extract with great blood glucose-balancing actions.

Bitter Melon: a botanical extract with great blood glucose-balancing actions.

Fenugreek: a botanical extract with great blood glucose-balancing actions.

Bilberry: a botanical extract with powerful antioxidant and sight-preserving actions.

Vanadium: a key trace mineral required for blood glucose balance.

Table 5: Nutrients in Doctor's Choice for Diabetics

Amount per two tablets:

Vitamin C (ascorbic acid)	300 mg
Vitamin E (as mixed tocopherols)	100 IU
Vitamin B6 (as pyridoxine HCL)	10 mg
Folic Acid	400 mcg
Vitamin B12 (as cyanocobalamin)	400 mcg
Biotin	1 mg
Magnesium (as chelated with citrate, fumarate, malate, succinate and alpha-ketoglutarate)	100 mg
Zinc (as zinc picolinate)	7.5 mg
Selenium (as L-selenomethionine)	50 mcg
Copper (as copper gluconate)	0.5 mg
Manganese (as chelated with citrate, fumarate, malate, succinate and alpha-ketoglutarate)	3.5 mg
Chromium (as chromium picolinate)	200 mcg
Sodium	20 mcg
Gymnema (gymnema sylvestre) Leaf Extract standardised to contain 25 per cent gymnemic acids	200mg

Bitter melon (nomardica charantia) Fruit Extract	200 mg
Fenugreek (trigonella foenum-graecum)	100 mcg
Bilberry (vaccinium myrtillus) Berry Extract	
standardised to contain 25 per cent anthocyanosides	
calculated as anthocyanidins	40 mg
Mixed Bioflavonoids 50 per cent (from citrus fruits)	25 mg
Vanadium (from 5 mg Vanadyl sulfate)	1.6 mg

Other ingredients: cellulose, modified cellulose gum, modified cellulose, titanium dioxide colour, lecithin and carnauba. Contains no sugar, wheat, gluten, corn, dairy products, artificial flavouring or preservatives. All colours used are from natural sources.

Doctor's Choice for Diabetics is safe for all diabetics to use and can be combined safely with injected insulin or oral hypoglycaemic drugs. The recommended dosage is two tablets taken twice daily with meals. This has, indeed, been a great help to me, as has *Dia-Comp*, which provides vitamins and minerals vital for optimal blood sugar regulation and carbohydrate metabolism, combined with herbs chosen specifically for their balancing effects on blood glucose levels. It contains:

Gymnema sylvestre, which has long been used for improving blood glucose control in diabetics. Components of *gymnema*, such as gymnemic acid, block the sensation of sweetness when applied to the tongue and, in clinical studies, this has resulted in the subjects consuming fewer calories at a meal. It is thought that *gymnema* enhances the production of endogenous insulin through regeneration of the insulin-producing pancreatic beta cells. When Type II diabetics were given *gymnema* alongside their oral hypoglycaemic drugs, 21 out of 22 subjects were able to considerably reduce their drug dosage and five subjects were able to discontinue their medication and maintain blood sugar control with *gymnema* extract alone. (*See* Baskaran, K. et al., 'Anti-diabetic effect of a leaf extract of *gymnema sylvestre* in non-insulin-dependent diabetes mellitus patients', in *J Ethnopharmacol* (1990), pp. 301–06).

Bitter Melon has been shown to exert a blood sugar-lowering action in human clinical trials. It is composed of several compounds with anti-diabetic properties, including charantia, a hypoglycaemic agent. In trials with Type II diabetic patients, oral administration of *Bitter Melon* preparations significantly improved glucose tolerance, reduced postprandial blood sugar levels and even decreased glycosylation haemoglobin levels in several patients. (*See* Srivastava, Y. et al., 'Anti-diabetic and adaptogenic properties of momordica charantia extract; an experimental and clinical evaluation', in *Phytother Res* (1986) 7, pp. 282–422.)

Fenugreek Seed Extract has demonstrated anti-diabetic effects in experimental and clinical studies, reducing fasting blood sugar and improving glucose tolerance levels. It has also been shown to decrease blood LDL, VLDL, and trigylceride levels whilst raising HDL.

Table 6: Nutrients in Dia-Comp

Two capsules contain:

Vitamin E (mixed tocopherols)	50 IU
Magnesium chelate	100 mg
Vitamin C (ascorbic acid)	100 mg
Vitamin B6 (pyridoxine HCI)	10 mg
Manganese (chelate)	10 mg
Zinc picolinate	5 mg
Biotin	1,000 mcg
Vitamin B12 (cyanocobalamin)	250 mcg
Chromium picolinate	50 mcg
Selenium (aspartate)	40 mcg
Blueberry extract (vaccinium myrtillus fructus)	300 mg
Gymnema Sylvestre extract standardised to contain 24 per cent gymnemic acid	150 mg
Bitter Melon extract (momordica charantia)	100 mg
Fenugreek Seed extract (trigonella foenum graecum)	100 mg

Contains no sugar, salt, yeast, wheat, gluten, corn, dairy products, colouring, flavouring or preservatives.

Recommended dosage is two capsules three times daily as an addition to the everyday diet. It has no known side effects when taken at the stated dose.

Another helpful alternative is *Bioactive B12*, which contains methylcobalamin, the active form of vitamin B12 (cobalamin). It exerts benefits well beyond those of other forms of vitamin B12 – it is delivered far better to nerve tissues, where it functions in accelerating transmethylation reactions in the manufacture of nucleic acids, neurotransmitters and phospholipids. As well as being of use as a dietary supplement for sufferers of diabetic retinopathy (a potentially blinding complication of diabetes), *Bioactive B12* may be of particular use for vegetarians and vegans, whose diets can be lacking in B12. It may also benefit the elderly, asthmatics and sufferers of multiple sclerosis, tinnitus, low sperm counts and depression.

Each tablet contains 1,000 mcg of vitamin B12 (methylcobalamin) in a base of black cherry flavouring. It contains no sugar, salt, yeast, wheat, corn, soy, dairy products, colouring or preservatives.

As a recommended dose, dissolve one tablet under the tongue daily as an addition to the everyday diet. There are no known side effects.

Often, diabetics have to pay particular attention to their eyes (remember the endocrine system, where the adrenals and kidneys are involved) and must control their blood pressure especially carefully to help avoid retinopathy. However, the eyes can be greatly improved by *Bilberry Extract*. The macula, located in the centre of the retina, is the part of the eye responsible for good vision. Degeneration of the macula is the leading cause of severe visual loss in the United Kingdom, the rest of Europe and the United States, in people of 55 or older. It is thought that highly destructive molecules called free radicals may initiate the macular damage, and a reduction in the blood supply to the macula may exacerbate the degenerative process. Free radical damage can be prevented by antioxidants, including flavonoids, found in bilberries. These flavonoids help to maintain healthy capillary membranes, so they may be beneficial for sufferers of macular degeneration, diabetic retinopathy and night blindness. Indeed, scientific studies have shown that bilberry extract, when taken by healthy subjects, improves night vision, allows the eyes to adjust more quickly to darkness and to recover faster after exposure to glare.

Each tablet contains 80 mg of bilberry extract (vaccinium myrtillus fructus), standardised to contain 25 per cent anthocyanosides (20 mg) calculated as anthocyanidins. It contains no sugar, salt, yeast, wheat, corn, soy, dairy products, colouring, flavouring or preservatives.

The recommended dosage is one or two capsules three times a day as an addition to the everyday diet. There are no known side effects.

An even better remedy, very helpful if a diabetic's sight is deteriorating, is *Vision Essentials. Vision Essentials* contains ingredients essential for eye function, including vitamins A, C and B2 (riboflavin), with bilberry extract. Vitamins A and C are antioxidants. Riboflavin helps regenerate antioxidants after they have neutralised free radicals. The bilberry extract is standardised for its content of anthocyanosides, flavonoid compounds that have natural antioxidant activity.

Table 7: Nutrients in Vision Essentials

Essential Vitamins:

Vitamin A (beta-carotene)	5,000 IU
(non-toxic form of Vitamin A)	
Vitamin C (ascorbic acid)	100 mg
Riboflavin (vitamin B2)	5 mg

Other ingredients:

Bilberry extract (vaccinium myrtillus fructus)	80 mg
(standardised to contain 25 per cent anthocyanosides (20 mg per capsule) calculated as anthocyanidins)	

It contains no sugar, salt, yeast, wheat, corn, soy, dairy products, colouring, flavouring or preservatives.

VISION ESSENTIALS AND THE MAINTENANCE OF EYE HEALTH

Vision Essentials is a popular supplement for those wishing to maintain optimal eye health. It contains vitamin A (beta-carotene), an essential nutrient for the maintenance of mucous membranes and general eye functions, vitamin C, which is required for repair to the tissues of the eye, and vitamin B2, which is vital for light adaptation. It is found in the pigment of the retina and deficiencies in vitamin B2 may cause excess sensitivity to light and blurring of vision and the eyes may become easily tired. *Bilberry Extract* has been shown to improve night-time visual acuity, quicker adjustment to darkness and faster restoration of visual acuity after exposure to glare. Indeed, Second World War Royal Air Force pilots reported improved night-time visual acuity on bombing raids after consuming bilberries!

VISION ESSENTIALS AND CONTACT LENS WEARERS

Contact lens wearers often complain of increased dryness, irritation and tiredness of the eyes. *Vision Essentials* may help to prevent dryness by maintaining the health of the mucous membranes, soothing and maintaining the health of the eye tissues. Vitamin B2 also helps prevent tiredness.

VISION ESSENTIALS AND MACULAR DEGENERATION

The macula is located in the centre of the retina and is important for good vision. Macular degeneration is thought to be a leading cause of severe visual loss in people over 55 in Europe and the United States. It is thought that highly destructive molecules, called free radicals, may initiate the macular damage and a reduction in the blood supply to the macula may exacerbate the degenerative process. Free radical damage can be prevented by antioxidants, including carotenoids, such as beta-carotene and vitamin C plus flavonoids found within bilberries. Antioxidants act to neutralise free radicals and vitamin B2 helps to regenerate the antioxidants after they have carried out the neutralisation process. Blood supply to the macula can also be improved by the flavonoids found within bilberries, as they act to support healthy capillaries.

VISION ESSENTIALS AND DIABETICS

Vision Essentials helps to prevent the complications of diabetes on eye health, including diabetic retinopathy. The proanthocyanidins, a flavonoid sub-group found within bilberries, act to maintain healthy capillary membranes and vitamins A and C act to prevent degeneration of the eye tissues due to free radical damage.

VISION ESSENTIALS AND CATARACTS

The antioxidant components of *Vision Essentials* also help to prevent the formation of cataracts, or can prevent any advancement of existing cataracts. Studies on vitamin B2 have also shown that this vitamin may be beneficial in cataract prevention.

VISION ESSENTIALS AND NIGHT BLINDNESS

The proanthocyanidin flavonoids found within bilberries, combined with vitamin B2 in *Vision Essentials*, have been found to improve night-time visual acuity in individuals suffering from night blindness.

IP-6 AND *INOSITOL*

New research suggests that *IP-6* and *inositol* may play a key role in insulin production.

Background

Diabetes is a disease in which insulin is not released in sufficient quantities (hence the requirement for injections in Type I diabetes) due to failure of the beta cells of the pancreas. In this case, blood sugars can elevate out of control and not enter the body's cells efficiently enough for normal energy production, causing a variety of symptoms ranging from increased thirst and urinary frequency through to confusion, stupor and coma in severe cases. Type I diabetes is also associated with degenerative changes in eyes, cardiovascular and renal systems. In early cases of Type II diabetes, insulin may be produced, but the body's cells fail to respond to it in the normal way. There appears to be a problem in the way the cell insulin receptors react to insulin and the glucose receptors react to glucose. As the condition progresses, insulin production appears to reduce. For most sufferers, dietary control can adequately manage the problem but Type II patients can suffer similar long-term side effects to Type I. However, they are far less likely to experience confusion, stupor and coma, as long as they balance their diet.

The development of IP-6

Inositol hexaphosphate (IP-6) and related inositol phosphates are abundant in the body. They act to regulate many cell processes, ranging from normal cell division associated with all living tissue through to the molecular control of complex cellular chemistry. It is this body-wide action that interested Prof. Shamsuddin, MD, PhD, University of Maryland and author of *IP-6: Nature's Revolutionary Cancer-Fighter* (Kensington, 1998) and prompted his in-depth study of the role of *IP-6* in colon cancer. During his research, he discovered other interesting side effects of *IP-6* that, at the time, appeared to be unrelated. As time passed, it became clear that the growth-regulating and anti-cancer effects of *IP-6* occurred by virtue of its interaction with many cellular processes that used *IP-6* as an intermediate substance in a long and complex control process. Without *IP-6*, many of these biological processes were unable to continue beyond a certain point which, in the case of cancer, could be seen as a failure of certain tissues to stop growing and dividing when mutations occurred. In other words, an *IP-6*-dependent cellular checking mechanism had failed and damaged, or genetically mutated cells were allowed to multiply unchecked to form a tumour. This discovery soon helped to answer how *IP-6* helped those with other non-cancer-related diseases, such as kidney stones, heart disease, sickle cell anaemia and, more recently discovered, diabetes.

IP-6 *and diabetes – simple observation and the latest science*

Some time ago, a colleague of Prof. Shamsuddin reported on some clinical follow-ups involving six or seven patients (himself included) with Type II diabetes and noted that the requirement for hypoglycaemic drugs went down, and that an acceptable blood glucose level was maintained whilst they were taking the *IP-6* and *inositol* product. At the time, Prof. Shamsuddin considered that this observation occurred as a result of altered glucose metabolism. Using established knowledge, he commented that the cellular level of *inositol* and *IP-3* goes down in diabetes and that by taking *IP-6* and *inositol* (which do *not* require insulin to get inside the cell), the levels of *IP-6* could be replenished. The depleted supply of *IP-3* can be increased by taking the *IP-6* and *inositol* combination, since *IP-6* combines with the *inositol* and is rapidly converted into a plentiful supply of *IP-3* once inside the body. By normalising the *IP-3* levels within the body's cells, it was thought, any defective mechanisms that relied on *IP-3* were corrected, resulting in improved blood glucose metabolism and, therefore, less dependence on hypoglycaemic drugs. This theory now appears to be supported by a new line of research published in December 2002 in the *American Journal of Physiology*. Scientists recognised the importance of the interactions that occur between glucose and the body's cells. If these interactions were defective, insulin production could not be triggered properly, nor could insulin, once released, regulate further insulin being unnecessarily released. This feedback mechanism is at the core of the diabetes problem, which is one of lost glucose–insulin regulation. *Inositol hexaphosphate* (*IP-6*) and its related substance (*IP-3*) have now been shown to be the key to this regulatory process. By keeping the cell levels of *IP-3* up (by taking *IP-6* and *inositol* on a daily basis) the cells' communication system between glucose and insulin can be radically improved. This process, known as signal transduction, appears to bring the beta cells of the pancreas back to life and retunes the body's tissues to the effects of insulin once again. This has obvious and widespread implications on the management of diabetes, a condition that, once diagnosed, carried the prognosis of a lifetime's commitment to medication and a strict dietary regime.

The story of *IP-6* and diabetes highlights the importance of both science and simple observation. What could be considered as an interesting effect or coincidence relating to taking *IP-6* and *inositol* supplements can now be explained by hard science. Many other interesting observations revolving around this key cell regulator await their baptism by science but, until that time, it would appear to be safe to allow science to catch up eventually with the clinical observations!

An article by Dr Michael T. Murray, an American naturopath, states that *IP-6* and *inositol* were discovered as nature's revolutionary cancer fighters. One of the hottest nutritional products to be introduced in years is the combination of *IP-6* and *inositol*. This combination of naturally occurring compounds produced from rice bran has demonstrated impressive anti-cancer and immune-enhancing effects in experimental studies.

What exactly is IP-6?
IP-6 is a component of fibre that is found primarily in whole grains and legumes. It appears that the cancer-protective effects of a high-fibre diet are due to the presence of higher levels of *IP-*

6 in the fibre. However, although *IP-6* is found in substantial amounts in the fibre component of whole grains and beans, supplementation with purified *IP-6* and the proper amount of *inositol* offers several advantages. First of all, in grains and beans, the *IP-6* exists primarily as a poorly absorbed form because it is complexed with protein and minerals like calcium, magnesium or potassium to form a salt. So, in its natural state as a fibre component, *IP-6* is poorly absorbed. Studies have shown that pure *IP-6* is significantly more bioavailable (or better absorbed) than the *IP 6* found in whole grains and beans. Furthermore, *IP-6* is rapidly taken up by cancer cells. This action is important as *IP-6* exerts significant beneficial effects within cancer cells basically, it turns cancer cells off (this effect will be discussed in more detail below).

Why should I take IP-6 *if I eat a high-fibre diet?*

Diabetics should certainly continue to eat a high-fibre diet, but supplementing the diet with *IP-6* and *inositol* provides substantially greater protection. Let's take a look at a study conducted at the University of Maryland. The study investigated whether a high-fibre diet would be as effective as pure *IP-6* in fighting cancer. Three groups of rats were studied. Group one was the control group; they simply ate standard 'rat food'. Group two was fed up to 20 per cent of their diet as wheat bran. Group three was given the equivalent amount of *IP-6* as the bran-supplemented group, only in the pure form. Compared to the control group, after 29 weeks rats fed up to 20 per cent bran had only an 11.4 per cent reduction in the number of tumours. However, rats given the pure *IP-6* at a level equal to that amount provided in the 20 per cent bran group had a nearly 50 per cent reduction in the number of tumours. In other words, pure *IP-6* as a supplement was at least four times more effective than a high-fibre diet. Put into human terms, these numbers translate to significantly greater protection being offered by pure *IP-6* than a high-fibre diet.

Why is pure IP-6 so much more effective than a high-fibre diet in reducing cancer?

The explanation was given above, but Dr Murray explains it again slightly differently. In whole fibre or bran, or cereals, *IP-6* is bound to the protein in a complex form. To be able to be absorbed and transported to the various organs and sites of cancer or potential trouble spots, *IP-6* must first be released from the protein complexes. It is often very difficult for the body to break down these *IP-6* protein complexes. So, even though a high-fibre diet may have high levels of *IP-6*, not all of it is available for absorption. Pure *IP-6* provides much better protection because more of it gets absorbed – it is more bioavailable.

Why is IP-6 *combined with inositol?*

This remarkable combination was discovered by Prof. Shamsuddin. *Inositol*, a member of the B-vitamin family, dramatically increases the anti-cancer and immune-enhancing effects of *IP-6*. Prof. Shamsuddin discovered that when properly combined with *inositol*, *IP-6* forms two molecules of *IP-3* in the body. *Inositol*, the backbone structure of *IP-6*, has six carbon atoms that are capable of binding phosphate molecules; when all six carbons are occupied by six phosphate groups, it forms *IP-6*. When only three of the carbons are bound by phosphate it is called *IP-3*. This chemistry is important because, although *IP-6* is gaining all the attention, it is really *IP-3* that is doing all the work. *IP-3* plays an important role inside the cells of our bodies. It basically functions as an on/off switch for human cancers, according to experimental studies in cell cultures. When *IP-3* levels are low (as in cancer cells), the cells replicate out of control. That basically is what occurs in cancer. When cancer cells are bathed in a broth of *IP-3*, they literally turn themselves off. This action reflects the central role that *IP-3* plays in controlling key cell functions, including replication and the communication between cells. Prof. Shamsuddin has discovered the proper ratio of *IP-6* and *inositol* to ensure the formation of *IP-3* within the body.

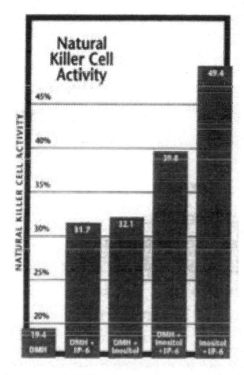

When *IP-6* combines with *inositol*, they are converted into two molecules of *IP-3* within the body.

What effect does the combination of* IP-6 *and* inositol *have on the immune system?

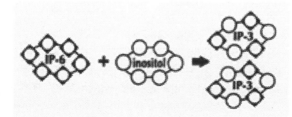

The combination of *IP-6* and *inositol* has also been shown to be an effective antioxidant and booster of immune function. The combination is especially helpful in boosting the activity of a type of white blood cell known as a 'natural killer', or 'NK' cell. These natural killer cells get their name because they literally kill cancer cells, viruses and other infecting organisms. They play a major role in protecting the body against cancer and infection. While *IP-6* alone can boost NK cell activity, the combination exerts even greater enhancement.

What about anti-cancer effects?

Based upon extensive experimental studies in animals and cell cultures, the combination of *IP-6* and *inositol* exerts anti-cancer effects against virtually all types of cancers, including cancers of the breast, prostate, lung, skin and brain, as well as in lymphomas and leukaemia. Table 8 lists some of the cancer cell lines that *IP-6* has shown activity against.

Table 8: Cancer and IP-6

Tissue or Organ Type	Cell Line
Brain Tumour	SR.B10A
Breast Cancer	MCF-7, MDA-MB-231 & -435
Colon Carcinoma	HT-29
Fibroblast, Immortalised	BALBc-3T3
Leukaemia	K-562, HL-60
Liver Carcinoma	Hep G2
Lung Carcinoma	HTB-119, RTE
Prostate Carcinoma	PC-3
Skeletal Muscle Sarcoma	RD
Skin Carcinoma	JB6

How does IP-6 work to fight cancer?

In addition to its antioxidant and immune-enhancing effects, *IP-6* exerts a number of interesting anti-cancer actions. Prof. Shamsuddin believes that the central pathway of *IP-6* action involves taking control of cell division. Cancer cells are out of control, dividing uncontrollably. What *IP-6* does in the cancer cell is literally turn off the switch that is telling the cell to divide. Prof. Shamsuddin and others have shown that *IP-6* reduces the rate of cancer cells in both animal and cancer cell studies by reducing the manufacture of new DNA (the genetic code). Since it does not exert the same inhibition in normal cells, *IP-6* is dramatically different from conventional anti-cancer agents. Chemotherapy drugs, for example, work by literally killing cells rather indiscriminately and, as a result, are quite toxic because they are killing the good cells as well as the bad. *IP-6* is dramatically different because it helps the cell to function normally, without damaging healthy cells.

And the combination of IP-6 and inositol is more powerful than IP-6 alone?

Yes. Prof. Shamsuddin has proven that the combination exerts much greater effect than *IP-6* alone. This has been demonstrated in animal models for breast cancer, lung cancer and colon cancer. For example, let's take a look at the study of colon cancer prevention. In this study, mice were given a compound (DMH) to induce cancer formation. Of these, one group was additionally treated with *IP-6*, another group with *inositol*, another with a combination of *IP-6* and *inositol*. The results indicate that the mice treated with *IP-6* alone or *inositol* alone had lower occurrences of tumours per animal. This benefit was greatly enhanced when *IP-6* and *inositol* were given in combination. The table below (and the earlier graph) clearly illustrates the superiority of the combination.

Table 9: Effect of IP-6, inositol, and the combination of IP-6 and inositol on intestinal tumours in mice

	Tumour Prevalence*	Tumour Frequency**
DMH	63 per cent	116 per cent
DMH + *IP-6*	47 per cent	62 per cent
DMH + *inositol*	30 per cent	45 per cent

| DMH + IP-6 + *inositol* | 25 per cent | 25 per cent |
| Control | 0 per cent | 0 per cent |

* per cent of mice with tumours
** per cent of tumours per mouse

How much IP-6 and inositol should I take?

Prof. Shamsuddin recommends taking a daily dosage of 800–1,200 mg of *IP-6* along with 200–300 mg of *inositol* as a general preventative measure. In patients with cancer or those who are at high risk for cancer, Prof. Shamsuddin recommends a dosage of 4,800–7,200 mg of *IP-6* along with 1,200–1,800 mg of *inositol*. He also recommends that it be taken on an empty stomach.

What about safety?

IP-6 is extremely safe, based upon extensive animal testing and human studies. In fact, no side effects have been reported even at higher dosages. You could not ask for a safer nutritional product.

Can IP-6 and inositol be used along with conventional cancer treatments?

Absolutely. Studies have shown that this combination can be used with conventional cancer treatments such as radiation and chemotherapy. In fact, according to Prof. Shamsuddin, *IP-6* and *inositol* have been shown to potentiate these therapies.

How do I know if I am taking an effective combination of IP-6 and inositol?

Look for products that contain a 4:1 ratio of *IP-6* to *inositol* for maximum benefit.

Where can I learn more about IP-6 and inositol?

Prof. Shamsuddin's book, *IP-6: Nature's Revolutionary Cancer-Fighter* (Kensington, 1998), is highly recommended. It can be found in good bookshops and health-food stores.

Summary

Description: The combination of *IP-6* and *inositol* is derived from rice bran and is an important intracellular regulator in human cells.

Actions: Enhances natural killer cell activity; protects against cancer; decreases proliferation of cancerous cells; antioxidant.

What to look for: A combination product that contains a 4:1 ratio of *IP-6* to *inositol.*

How much to take: For prevention: 800–1,200 mg *IP-6* and 200–300 mg *inositol.* For cancer patients: 4,800–7,200 mg *IP-6* and 1,200–1,800 mg *inositol.*

As I have said before, cancer and diabetes are both metabolic diseases, so they have something in common. During the research into this product, it was discovered by chance that not only is it of terrific help with cancer patients, but it also plays a key role in insulin production and in the management of diabetes. I have therefore now introduced *inositol* into my own daily diet. To my great surprise it has been of tremendous help; I have found the great benefits of this extra alternative remedy such a worthwhile discovery.

DETOXIFICATION

I wouldn't be a real naturopath if I didn't say a little on detoxification. The lymphatic system, which works during the night and mops up the waste material in the body, needs you to have plenty of sleep, but also needs some thorough liver and blood cleansing. Detoxification processes are of great benefit, and one of the finest of them all is the Detox Box from Alfred Vogel. Alfred Vogel and I put this box together many years ago. It is a spring-cleaning course for the gall bladder, liver, bowel, kidneys and stomach, and also starts off the detoxification of the lymphatic system. In 24 hours, the liver filters 1,200 pints of blood and can benefit from some help. It has a few real enemies (nicotine, alcohol and too much animal fat) and a few very good friends (one of which is oxygen). To enable the liver to carry out its work properly, detoxification is necessary. Artichokes are also very beneficial, as too is *milk thistle*.

Dr Megan Shields MD writes that *milk thistle phytosome* gives superior protection in a toxic world. Every day we are exposed to a barrage of environmental pollutants – industrial chemicals, pesticides and nuclear radiation, not to mention preservatives, synthetic hormones and other veterinary drugs in packaged foods and in meat. A wide range of contaminants is also found in cosmetics and household cleaning products. More than 100 different toxic chemicals have been found stored in human fat. Yet this is only the tip of the iceberg when it comes to our exposure to toxic chemicals on a daily basis. Many toxins are eliminated from the body, leaving no trace of their presence – but only after they've damaged our health.

The consequences of exposure to toxins can be minimised thanks to the liver. The liver is responsible for detoxifying and filtering more than a litre of blood per minute, in addition to its other functions, including:

- Breaking down the body's own natural hormones, such as oestrogen and cortisols
- Producing secretions, such as bile for digestion
- Playing a critical role in carbohydrate, fat and protein metabolism, as well as storage of vitamins

However, the liver won't be able to perform its many essential, wide-ranging functions, necessary to health, if it has been damaged by an onslaught of toxic chemicals, bacterial invaders, alcohol abuse or even some over-the-counter and prescription drugs (ranging from acetaminophen to birth-control pills).

As a family practitioner and detoxification expert, Dr Shields has treated several thousand people for both acute and low-level chemical exposure. Her patients have included painters and decorators, artists, firemen, farm workers, families exposed to fumigation chemicals, people whose drinking water was contaminated with solvents, factory workers, people exposed to toxic chemicals in their carpeting, children exposed to radiation and, unfortunately, increasing numbers of people who are addicted to recreational drugs or those prescribed by well-meaning doctors.

Particularly in the area of protective nutrients, fortunately *milk thistle* is excellent for helping people deal with toxic overload. This herbal powerhouse, which blends nature's own powerful healing nutrients with cutting edge science and technology, in Shields' words has quickly become recognised as 'the Cadillac of liver protectants'. It is available in health food stores.

This natural miracle healer has long been used to treat liver disorders and is one of the most thoroughly scientifically validated plant extracts. Anyone who grew up using recreational drugs or living in urban or other areas of chemical pollution – in fact, anybody living in this modern chemical world – would benefit from the use of *milk thistle*. People should also use *milk thistle* if they have been diagnosed with a condition such as congested liver (inadequate bile flow), cirrhosis (a degenerative, inflammatory condition in which the liver cells harden, caused by excess alcohol intake), or hepatitis (liver inflammation and enlargement).

A true story relayed by Dr Shields illustrates the importance of *milk thistle* for anyone who has suffered a chemical exposure or who has a liver condition. In 1991, her colleague, Cynthia Watson, MD, a skilled herbal healer from Santa Monica, CA, faced one of the greatest challenges of her professional career. She was called upon to treat 20 men and women, victims of a pesticide poisoning episode that occurred in the small Californian tourist town of Dunsmuir. A train derailment caused the spill of thousands of gallons of a highly toxic rice pesticide, metam sodium. Sixty miles of the upper Sacramento River were polluted with virtually all life disappearing – from insects to deer and bear. The human toll was also tragic. Many of the local people, who had received emergency medical treatment at local hospitals, had gone from specialist to specialist, but were still sick with headaches, fever, nausea, vomiting, muscle aches, impotence, memory loss and other signs of acute chemical exposure, including significant liver damage. A clinical faculty instructor at the University of Southern California, Dr Watson treated many of her patients with high-quality extracts of *milk thistle*. One of her patients, Wayne Cunningham, a barge operator who was asked to operate pumping and dispersing equipment at the headwaters of Lake Shasta as the spill worked its way down river, was extremely ill. He credits *milk thistle* with saving his life.

We don't know all the reasons why *milk thistle* is so helpful to the liver, even when it is under severe toxic stress. But we do know that it stimulates the liver's production of antioxidants, helping prevent further damage. It also builds up the levels of glutathione, a small, protein-based molecule that helps the body metabolise pesticides and other environmental toxins. According to research from the September 1996 issue of the *Journal of Pharmacy and Pharmacology*, we have learned that *milk thistle* also has anti-inflammatory effects. *Milk thistle* stimulates protein synthesis, causing enhanced production of new liver cells to replace those that have been damaged.

The list of studies on *milk thistle*'s liver-production benefits is long and convincing. Its place in the *materia medica* of natural healing is safely assured.

SUPER *MILK THISTLE*!

Imagine what would happen if we could enhance the bioavailability of *milk thistle*! That's precisely what a team of European scientists set out to do. Researchers have learned how to combine the active ingredient in *milk thistle*, silybin, with phosphatidylcholine to create a compound known as a phytosome that is highly absorbable by the body. This greatly enhances the body's ability to use the healing nutrients found in *milk thistle*. This *milk thistle* extract has been proven to provide even better healing effects. In a 1992 report in the *Japanese Journal of Pharmacology*, this new compound was compared with ordinary silybin in an animal experiment, and it was found to be far more effective in preventing liver damage. In fact, it showed a 'significant . . . protective activity' against a wide range of assaults on the liver.

Other studies also confirm superior benefits from *milk thistle phytosome*. A 1991 report in *Planta Medica* noted that *milk thistle phytosome*'s availability in the body 'is several-fold greater' than its unbound counterpart. An experimental study, reported in 1992 in the *European Journal of Drug Metabolism and Pharmacokinetics*, indicates a 'superior bioavailability'. Clearly, the evidence supports *milk thistle extract phytosome* as the best form available.

A nineteenth-century tincture was first made with *milk thistle* seeds, *Tinctura Cardui Mariae Rademacher*. It is still listed in modern medical drug references. Then came the identification of one of the actual active principles, silybin, which allowed for standardisation and enhanced effects. Now comes the next generation: *milk thistle phytosome*. *Milk thistle* is good, make no mistake. *Milk thistle phytosome* is better.

If you want the very best *milk thistle* product, use the following guidelines:

- It should be bound with phosphatidylcholine
- It should be standardised to contain 80 per cent silymarin calculated as silybin, the compound in silymarin that yields the greatest degree of biological activity
- It should be formulated with highest-quality liver-supporting nutrients, including extracts of dandelion, artichoke and liquorice root

WHO NEEDS MILK THISTLE?

Those with the following health-related factors in their lives should seriously consider regular supplementation with *milk thistle phytosome*:

- History of liver disease
- Consume alcohol
- Use medically prescribed or recreational drugs
- Use over-the-counter drugs
- Work in an industry where toxic chemical exposure
  is common
- Live near agricultural activity where pesticides are used
- Chemically sensitive
- History of toxic exposures

GET THE TOXINS OUT OF YOUR DIET

Eating lower on the food web is a good way to reduce your exposure to environmental toxins and reduce the stress on your liver. Many of the most toxic chemicals in the diet, such as DDT and heptachlor, as well as radiation, are found in their highest concentrations in 'red light' foods such as beef and dairy. If you are health-conscious, diabetic or not, you should make sure when you do choose to consume these foods that they are natural or organic. This means the animals were raised without veterinary drugs, including antibiotics and hormones, and fed grains grown without pesticides.

Be sure to eat organic vegetables, fruit and grains whenever possible. These substantially reduce exposure to environmental toxins because they are not contaminated with pesticides and because they provide fibre which helps absorb and transport toxins from the body. Also avoid processed foods, especially products with unsafe additives, such as aspartame, saccharin and artificial colours.

DETOX WITH EXERCISE

Being a couch potato has become a way of life. Yet, as Dr Shields confirms, exercise is highly protective against environmental toxins. In experimental studies, she states that animals that exercise the most have the greatest resistance to the effects of cancer-causing chemicals. So regular exercise is extremely important. Besides, one of the body's most important methods of natural detoxification is through perspiration. In Shields' clinical work in the area of detoxification, a number of lab reports have been reviewed from patients that clearly show we literally 'sweat out' toxins, from drugs to heavy metals and pesticides.

Purchase safe cleaning products and take other measures to eliminate toxic inputs to the home environment. 'Instead of furniture polish with petroleum distillates, plain mineral or vegetable oil with vitamin E as a preservative works well too,' advises Michael Wisner, co-author of *Living Healthy in a Toxic World* (Perigee, 1996). 'Instead of mothballs which contain naphthalene, a nerve and reproductive toxin, use cedar blocks and chips. Avoid plastic or galvanised plumbing – copper is preferred. Avoid using urea-formaldehyde foam or fibreglass insulation. Both chemicals are cancer-causing.'

Dr Shields is convinced that it is possible to stay healthy in today's environment, but that our bodies require significant help. Low toxin living is part of the answer, but for many people whose bodies require extra detoxification assistance, the use of a quality *milk thistle phytosome* supplement can also be an extremely important ally for healthy living.

A brighter future for diabetics has also been promised by recent research that suggests vitamin E may reduce the long-term risks of complications in diabetics. It was quite interesting to see that the five-time Olympic gold medallist, Sir Steve Redgrave CBE, is positive proof that diabetics can lead not only normal lives but extraordinary lives, full of vitality and enthusiasm. Fast-acting antioxidant protection is necessary and recent research has shown that vitamin E, in particular, may help to prevent the vascular problems associated with diabetes, even to the extent that peripheral neuropathy can be helped. Studies on vitamin E have shown the benefits that this vitamin can give, even if oxidative damage is involved in the vascular system of diabetics, so the improvement of antioxidant protection is very important. Vitamin deficiencies are often apparent in diabetic patients. Even though diabetes mellitus is said to be an incurable metabolic disease, some help is available.

In Type I diabetes the symptoms of frequent urination, fatigue and rapid loss of weight is an autoimmune disease that usually appears in people under 40. However, with the combination of *IP-6* and vitamin E improvements have been shown. Type II diabetes is the most common type, where the body no longer responds normally to its own insulin, and this can sometimes be helped with diet.

The latest report shows that in many countries diabetes is on the increase amongst young people. It is most interesting to see that the World Health Organisation estimates the number of diabetic patients worldwide has doubled in the last ten years and that up to 140 million people globally suffer from diabetes and this figure might double again by the year 2025. It is also interesting to see that diabetes is the main cause of blindness in adults and that the risk is ten times higher in diabetics than in healthy people. Diabetics also have a two- to four-fold higher risk of cardiovascular disease, which is the major cause of death in diabetic patients. Kidney failure, which affects up to one in three Type I diabetics, often results in dialysis or kidney transplantation. Complications involving the small blood vessels, kidney failure or need of amputation caused by the damage done and peripheral neuropathy (the disturbance of the peripheral nervous system) affects half of all diabetics. This often results in loss of sensation in the feet and legs and can end in amputation. The alternatives to insulin or drug-related products for diabetes are quite numerous, and it is worthwhile noting which alternatives are available, especially when problems surface if conventional methods fail. Sometimes in my practice, I have seen amazing results of diabetics who have come to the end of the road using conventional treatment and have been helped to recovery through alternative methods.

~ CHAPTER FOUR ~

What about the Emotions of a Diabetic?

A young doctor once told me that when he was working in a hospital and had to take the diabetes clinics, he found the patients very hard to deal with. He often found the diabetics difficult and, at times, unreasonable. I told him that over the years I have been dealing with diabetics, I have felt that it is not the diabetics themselves who are difficult, but that they are often misunderstood. One must not forget that wherever the endocrine system is involved the emotions play a big part. As I said in Chapter One, man has three bodies. Diabetes is greatly influenced by the third and most important body that man has – namely the emotional body. The endocrine system will be in harmony as long as each of the seven endocrine glands works well. If one is out of balance, then the others become imbalanced. It is therefore often very difficult to completely understand the emotional system of a diabetic and the large part it plays.

When I was younger, one of my aunts was diabetic. While I was studying, I stayed with her for quite a number of years and even after that, when we worked together, I often noticed the difficulty she had in accepting that she was diabetic. She often said that you get no sympathy when you have diabetes. She was probably correct, especially since diabetes was so misunderstood in the past. My aunt would say that she sometimes wished she had an illness where you could visibly see the symptoms because, as a diabetic, you mostly look well and therefore other people do not realise there is anything wrong with you. She was an insulin-dependent diabetic and in those days had to inject herself four times a day. It was a struggle, as she got upset very quickly; by nature she was sensitive and one had to be very careful in handling the situation. Mentally, she was not the strongest person, although she was intelligent. She certainly was greatly misunderstood, and had to do her utmost to balance her blood sugar. This often resulted in problems like comas, where she could suddenly collapse, completely unconscious, and this was aggravated by her mental state. In those days we called these episodes 'hypos' and my aunt sometimes had to be taken to hospital when they occurred.

I experienced some of the most severe diabetic symptoms with this aunt. Hypos were unknown in the small village hospital and therefore her diabetes caused great concern. Slowly more knowledge was gained on the subject and, as the years progressed, balancing her blood sugar became easier and she felt a bit better. I have never met a person who was so particular about her diet. I must say that she was determined to stick to a good healthy diet and would never touch anything that could even remotely contain sugar. Dietary management was absolutely essential in helping to balance her blood sugar. Her emotions, however, were very unpredictable. I do believe that the imbalance in her hormone system that had led to her diabetes contributed a lot to her mood swings, her emotions and the problems that arose, especially during the menopause, when things were extremely difficult for her.

The emotions of a diabetic must be understood and diabetics may need some guidance on how to balance them. I often think that the balance of the three bodies – physical, mental and emotional – needs what we call a holistic approach; we must treat not only the problems caused by the diabetes or the pancreas, but the whole body, so that they can work together. This reminds me of the many diabetics I have treated over the years and in particular of a woman who reminded me of my aunt. This particular lady had a great battle when she was young. She had discovered at a fairly early age that she was a lesbian and, therefore, was very misunderstood, as she was born and brought up in a very conservative farmer's family in the country. Not a lot was known about lesbians in her young days, at the beginning of the 1940s. She therefore had a great struggle with her conscience in order to overcome the misunderstanding and aggression focused towards her and, because of this, she gradually became very unwell. She then contracted a very nasty flu at the age of 18, which was so bad that she was hospitalised and, after various tests were carried out, she was finally diagnosed with diabetes. She struggled on in life but it was not until she was very much older that she started to accept her problems. Nevertheless, her diabetes was so bad that her health went from bad to worse and her life was one long strain. When she told me about her problems, I advised her to the best of my ability and, during the latter part of her life, things got much easier for her. It is because of this that I often emphasise that diabetes needs a lot of understanding.

Another young girl – whom I liked tremendously – comes to my mind. Because of the severity of her diabetes, she needed a lot of guidance. Her diabetes consultant was very understanding and, after she came to me, we worked together to help her – and she luckily improved greatly. Her kidneys were badly affected, hence the fluctuations in her blood pressure. Her immune system was also low because of these problems and she often suffered from colds, flus and infections. She was a very brave person who was never moody or difficult, but accepted her condition most graciously. We often talked to each other and I continued to offer her encouragement. She would never forget her daily injections and kept strictly to her diet. One thing I have learned with severe diabetics is that the quicker they get help when something goes wrong, the better. Unfortunately, one Christmas, when there was not much help available, she battled yet another problem and ended up in hospital. So often with diabetics, if one part of the body packs up, they all pack up, which was what happened in her case. Doctors and nurses fought hard to save her life but sadly, at the age of 28, her short life came to an end. I learned from that situation that with diabetes one has to be very careful – as I mentioned earlier, the seriousness of the condition should never be taken lightly. It is very important to get medical help as quickly as possible when things start to go wrong.

This reminds me of a lady who is now almost blind. She does not have as strong a will as the first two ladies I mentioned, and has a terrible battle with sugar. She often says, 'The spirit is willing, but the flesh is weak.' She simply cannot keep off Mars bars, chocolate and chocolate biscuits. She feels that she cannot cope if she doesn't have them. I have often told her that her kidneys are affected, her blood pressure is rising and she has nearly no sight left, yet she is completely unwilling to give up sugar. Her doctors, her diabetes nurse and I have pleaded with her, but she simply will not give them up. We often see in such cases that there is a psychological background to the problem and I have often talked to her about it, trying to find out what she is compensating for, as she has a wonderful home life and a most understanding husband. In fact, it has emerged that she had a very disturbed childhood. This can often be the case – not only with diabetics, but with everybody. You really need to get to the root of the problem, as emotions and mental attitude can attack the physical body to the extent that things become very serious.

I also learned from another young girl who, unfortunately, did not take her health seriously and died at a very young age. She entrusted a lot of her problems to me and talked about them often. She had a sort of bartering system – if I helped her with her diabetes, she would do as I asked to adjust her diet, as long as, some way or another, she could have some sugar. I often told her that that was impossible. I will never forget the day she finally decided that she would try to omit sugar from her diet, when she said, 'Please pray for me – I will start next week.' I asked, 'Why can you not start now? It is very important, because your blood sugar is very high and your injections will not help you if you do not keep to the dietary instructions of your dietician and the advice that I have given you.' She put a little medal in my hand and said, 'I shall do it from next week. I still want to enjoy myself this week.' These little bartering systems are so often very dangerous – that week this lovely young girl became very ill, landed up in hospital and died. I was very upset that I had not been forceful enough to get my message across to her and perhaps help to prevent her death.

We see too often that diabetics have strong minds and sometimes they are very determined in doing what they want and not what others advise. They convince themselves that they can do it their way and there will be no problem. This is often dangerous.

With pleasure, I think of a fairly severely diabetic gentleman who was under a lot of strain at work because of his high position and said to me, 'Yes, I will do what you say because I want to live. I don't want to pack it all in.' Although he depended greatly on his tablets, he too had problems, especially with alcohol, which I told him was probably the only thing that stopped him from getting his blood sugar towards six or seven, which he dearly wanted. He looked at me and said, 'I see that you mean it,' and I said, 'Absolutely.' He gave up alcohol that very same day and he has done so well that his doctor even advised him that he could come off his tablets. His diabetes is now completely dietary controlled. So, it can be done – it is possible if the diabetic makes up his or her mind to do it, and to stick to the rules which, in turn, will give him or her a much better life.

This reminds me of another young man who complained that he was so tired and sleepy – which of course can happen with diabetics – that he could hardly do his work. He was unwilling to give up smoking and drinking (which I advised him to do), but I convinced him to try for one week and, at the end of the week, to tell me how he felt. I asked him to make me a promise: 'If you feel a lot better, even after one week, can we make a deal that you give up the offenders, as I am sure that is what makes you so sleepy and unwell.' He made this promise, came back after a week and told me that he had never felt so well and that, after following my advice, he felt it would be worth giving up smoking and drinking in order to have a better life.

Of the many cases I have seen in my 45 years of practice, I am reminded of yet another young man who was a diabetic, but also under severe stress at work. His business was suffering, his marriage was suffering, he had become impotent and struggled just to exist. He became very unwell. Everyone tried their best to help. His wife was very understanding when he was so unwell, but he was really in the depths of despair. All of his three bodies were in great turmoil, yet somewhere there was a little flash of hope that he would get better. When he reached his lowest point, he made up his mind that if he got better, he would give up his business and fully adhere to the advice from his diabetes consultant and dietician, and would also follow my advice from a complementary position. His wife was distressed and asked me to see him. I went to the hospital and talked to him and encouraged him to fight his illness. He fought and he fought and when he felt he could not go on fighting much longer, the little flash of hope started to become brighter and brighter. Along with his wife, I helped him through this very dark period of his life. He came out of it feeling positive, with his marriage restored; he left behind all his business worries and found a job. It is with great happiness that I see this man with his wife from time to time in my consulting room, after having shared the worst experiences of his life, when he was very close to death.

Think how wonderfully the body works and study the endocrine system a little and you will realise why diabetics and emotions (which play such a very big part) need a lot of understanding. I have often found that diabetics, in particular, need a lot of explanations. They can be difficult people, but that is mostly because of the underlying cause of their emotional state. Explanation and dialogue for diabetics are very important; only then will diabetics understand that although they might often be emotional people, the harmony within the three bodies is of the greatest importance.

~ CHAPTER FIVE ~

What about Lifestyle?

Early one Saturday morning, a young businessman consulted me. He was in utter despair, the reason being that he had become a diabetic. He had a busy life, a beautiful wife, two children and a very successful business, but his diabetes had made him almost impotent. He said he felt that life was not worth living. Although he was young, he was very often tired, had lost interest in any sexual activity and felt he was on the verge of losing his wife.

As he was so despondent, I felt I had to allow additional time to talk to him and tried to reassure him that all was not lost. After listening to his story, I said that he should not blame everything on diabetes. I surmised that he put his business first by working day and night to establish it and that he devoted most of his time to work, and had gradually come to put his wife and family second. He nodded in agreement. He said he now had no family life, but still had a close relationship with his wife. I advised him that we would have to put everything in order. Firstly, his business was successful enough that he should be able to spend some time on himself and his family. I told him I would try to build up his energy and help him with his problems, not only in his family life but also with his impotence, which was a big problem for him.

He said that one of the things he enjoyed, when he had time, was to go out for a nice meal, but he didn't know how to tackle living without sugar and this caused him further difficulties. So I spoke to him about this first and, in simple terms, told him what diabetes really is, as he had never fully understood the disease. I told him that all was not lost and that if we worked methodically through his problems, I was sure it would all work out.

He had a very investigative mind and had been reading a lot on the subject. In fact, he asked me why the beta cells of the islets of Langerhans (the pancreatic islets) stop secreting the insulin needed to lower the sugar levels in blood, thus leading to raised blood sugar levels. I told him that several researchers had published the results of studies into the causes of diabetes to discover what it is that damages the beta cells and stops them from producing insulin. Interest had focused on one report of the existence of beta cell antibodies in the blood, and another showed that a drug called alloxan destroyed the pancreatic beta cells of mice injected with the drug, causing the mice to develop diabetes. There had also been speculation that excess production of oxygen radicals in the body may also be the cause. Combining these results and various other research papers on the topic, we can assume that a considerable percentage of diabetes cases, although not all, are aggravated by damage to the pancreatic beta cells from increases in oxygen radicals and lipid peroxides.

Therefore, diet is extremely important. He said he wasn't very keen on eating green vegetables, although he had read that green vegetables and some other foods mop up the free radicals, and he was particularly interested in that subject. I told him that free radicals are basically natural substances and that there are foods that can mop them up in the body. He then said, 'Well, if that means things like broccoli and spinach, I am not interested.' I agreed that these foods do include those vegetables, but told him that they also include salmon, tomatoes and that quite a number of other products would be effective. After that he became more interested.

Then he said that he really wanted to know what harm sugar and sugar products can do to the body, so I told him a bit about sugar and carbohydrates, and why there should be a balance between carbohydrates and protein. As he already had a few signs of atrophic tendencies, I told him the value of the acid-alkaline system and handed him a copy of my book, *The Ten Golden Rules for Good Health*, which is simply written to make it easier to understand a little bit of the very complex theories on the acid-alkaline system and the balance between carbohydrates and proteins. I told him that three things were interfering with his lifestyle: sugar, salt and stress. I also told him that because he was insulin-dependent, sugar was a poison. Sugar becomes a real problem when we use refined sugar regularly and, unfortunately, most people eat it without realising. For millions of people throughout the world, the sugar eaten comes not only from the sugar bowl, but is also hidden in a lot of foods. Producing sugar is a very lucrative business because people love to eat it. In the first place, as it is a highly concentrated substance, it is one of the best ways to preserve all kinds of foods because bacteria cannot live in it. Secondly, for some people, sugar is even more addictive than alcohol and nicotine. The list of products containing sugar is enormous. He then asked what people did in the olden days. I told him that 200 years ago, when people began to extract sugar from sugar beet, their palates became accustomed to sugar so quickly that they started to love the taste. Because of its manufacturing process, sugar became a lifeless substance which is damaging to health, not only with diabetes, but in many other ways. There was a time when science believed that diabetes had nothing to do with sugar. In some cases this is so, but with the overuse of sugar, the pancreas is under tremendous stress.

We then came to the probable reason why he had become impotent. I explained to him that sugar is a real thief of vitamins, minerals and trace elements. When sugar is manufactured, all the fibre, vitamins and minerals contained in the original product, the sugar beet, are discarded. However, the human organism cannot metabolise sugar or any other refined food when these vital substances are missing. Therefore, minerals and other vital substances have to be confiscated from the body's own reserves, which can be found, for example, in our teeth and bones. Even small children who eat many sweets and pastries will then suffer from dental decay.

For the same reason, many elderly people lose their teeth and, because of lack of exercise and bad eating habits, their bones become brittle and weak. Although nowadays in many homes for the elderly they serve a raw salad with or before the meal, coffee with a sweet dessert or a pastry is highly appreciated. This is a very bad custom, because refined sugar or flour in combination with raw salads will cause fermentation in the intestines, stomach-ache, flatulence and even more serious health problems.

The more sugar we eat, the greater becomes our lack of B vitamins, which are extremely important for our nerves. Nervous people and restless, sleepless children love sweets! While in a healthy body the metabolism of sugar from fruit, raw vegetables and cereals, which still contain all their original vital substances (vitamins, minerals, etc.), is never problematic, concentrated refined carbohydrates can be the cause of a sudden steep rise of the blood sugar level, called hyperglycaemia.

The pancreas produces insulin, needed for the assimilation of sugar. However, in the case of refined sugar, the pancreas produces far too much insulin. In nature, sugar is always combined with fibre, vitamins, minerals and other substances, so our pancreas still produces the quantity of insulin needed for the digestion of sugar cane or big sugar beets, instead of producing only the insulin needed for a small amount of sugar. After this sugar has been 'digested', there is still much insulin available, which should be used in some way. Now the craving for something sweet starts and, at the same time, the blood sugar level drops lower and lower. This condition is called hypoglycaemia and may cause extreme weakness, dizziness, fainting or even circulatory failure. The person affected thus will often go out of their way to obtain something sweet. As soon as, for example, they eat some chocolate, the craving abates, the level of the blood sugar goes up and everything is fine until the now-available sugar, in its turn, has been used. This can go on and on until a real addiction to sweets develops, which can be the cause of many serious diseases.

By treating this gentleman further – and I have seen him many times now – his life has returned to a normal, happy one. His impotence has disappeared and he has accepted his condition, especially once he realised that he wasn't alone and that help was available.

A vast increase in the number of people being diagnosed – especially with Type II diabetes – is a daily occurrence. In *Health Which?* of June 2002, Colin Meek wrote that the year 2015 will become pandemic with diabetes and, worryingly, that it will be particularly children who will be affected. I am not surprised by this statement, as I see the terrific use of sugar by children, and that chocolate butties – even worse than bacon butties – are becoming quite fashionable. The time bomb of diabetes is becoming a threat. About 1.4 million people in the UK have been diagnosed as having diabetes. Luckily, 85 per cent of those people have Type II as having Type I means that one is insulin-dependent. Type II is much more common and is usually diagnosed in older people. I am very happy to see that the NHS and the government are very concerned about these rising figures. Seven hundred and fifty million pounds has been put aside to be spent in carrying out more research into this enormous problem. It is of the utmost importance that people with diabetes look at their own diet, and that screening might be feasible to diagnose the illness early. It is at five minutes to twelve, not five minutes past twelve that action should be taken.

The fast-food industry needs to take a careful look at what it is doing to people's health – see my book, *Hidden Dangers in What We Eat and Drink*.

Steve Gillam from the King's Fund has said, 'We'll go on ignoring early disease signs and we won't provide optimal care to those who could benefit.' Prevention is better than cure. Diabetes, which is an enormous challenge for anyone working in healthcare, should be investigated thoroughly. One has to realise that diabetes is a serious and complex condition that affects many parts of the human body. If it is not controlled, it can cause heart disease, kidney disease, blindness and circulatory problems that might lead to amputation but, as I saw with this young, successful businessman, he used his common sense and listened to advice, and benefits today.

A serious look into one's lifestyle is very important. In addition to putting this gentleman on a healthy diet, I asked him to take two tablets of *Doctor's Choice for Diabetics*, twice a day. He also took *Molkosan* (one teaspoonful in half a cup of water, twice a day), which brought his weight down, and a fairly high dose of vitamin E, which I think is very important for diabetics. This has been a favourite for many sports people. Taking 400 IU, twice a day, can help control diabetes – just look at the Olympic rower and diabetic, Sir Steve Redgrave, CBE. Vitamin E can work as an antioxidant and is very helpful for vascular problems, which diabetic patients often have. It is crucial that preventative measures are taken after one is diagnosed with diabetes, when we often see tremendous vitamin deficiencies. Important studies conducted by several scientists and researched by the University of Naples examined the effects of vitamin E on oxidative stress and on the functioning of the nerves of the heart. Vitamin E very often, especially when there are vascular or blood circulatory problems, is of the greatest help.

One combination that I like to use with diabetics is Nature's Best *Vitamin E 400 IU with Selenium*. Its formula is:

Vitamin E d-Alpha Tocopheryl Succinate	269 mg (400 IU)
Selenium (as Seleno L-Methionine)	100 mg

Other ingredients: dicalcium phosphate, silicon dioxide, microcrystalline cellulose, magnesium stearate, stearic acid, crosslinked sodium carboxymethyl-cellulose and magnesium silicate.

The product is a combination of vitamin E, known for its role as an antioxidant, and selenomethionine, which contributes to the raw materials from which the body makes glutathione peroxidase, which also has an important antioxidant role in the body. Just as vitamins and minerals are often found to be naturally combined together in food sources, this product combines two nutrients with antioxidant properties. Selenomethionine is yeast free.

Dosage: One tablet daily with a meal, or as directed by practitioner.

Contraindications, warnings: Those suffering from hypertension should commence vitamin E supplementation gradually. Those on oral anticoagulants should be monitored.

Side Effects, over-usage: None known at the recommended usage.

I also find it very helpful to give *Zinc* (15 mg) from Nature's Best.
Each capsule of *Zinc* (as citrate) delivers:

Zinc (as citrate) 15 mg

Other ingredients: microcrystalline cellulose, gelatine, magnesium stearate and silicon dioxide.

Dosage: One capsule daily with a meal, or as directed by practitioner.

Each capsule of *Zinc* (as amino acid chelate) delivers:

Zinc (as amino acid chelate) 15 mg

Other ingredients: dicalcium phosphate, microcrystalline cellulose, crosslinked sodium carboxymethylcellulose, stearic acid and magnesium stearate.

Dosage: One tablet daily with a meal, or as directed by practitioner.

For this young man, these supplements were very helpful and I also prescribed some extra *Manpower*, a remedy from Michaels, which luckily helped him return to a normal sex life with his beloved wife. He became a happy man again; he is still very successful in business, but he got his priorities right and has become much more involved with his family.

Vitamins, minerals and trace elements are very important for a diabetic. Some of the remedies that are on the market nowadays are very helpful. It is very interesting to see, by looking into a diabetic's lifestyle, just what kind of problems can occur. Over the years, I have treated many diabetics and have naturally taken a special interest in this condition, being diabetic myself.

Because I am from a partially blind family on my mother's side, and because of my diabetes, I always take the greatest care by having regular eye tests. For those who begin to have loss of sight, especially patients who have Type I diabetes, dilated eye examinations and photographs are important. Early photographs are very helpful and, if the eyesight fails, I often prescribe *Vision Essentials* from Enzymatic Therapy, which, as mentioned earlier, includes bilberry extract, at the dose of one capsule taken twice a day. This usually works very well when taken in combination with some extra vitamin C. With diabetics in particular, I find that *Ester-C 500 mg capsules*, from Nature's Best, very helpful. Each capsule contains:

Vitamin C – 500 mg
(Vitamin C as calcium ascorbate and dehydroascorbic

acid, calcium C-metabolites, calcium carbonate, soya
lecithin and guar gum).

Other ingredients: microcrystalline cellulose, gelatine,
magnesium stearate and silicon dioxide.

Dosage: One to four capsules daily with a meal, or as directed
by practitioner.

Uses: *Ester-C* is a unique form of vitamin C, patented in the
USA. It is believed that *Ester-C* may be an improved form of the
vitamin. It has a neutral pH in solution, rendering it a very
gentle form of vitamin C which may be preferred by those who
suffer gastrointestinal symptoms when taking naturally acidic
forms of the vitamin.

Another problem that I have often encountered with Type II
diabetes is the risk of heart problems. This problem should be
treated properly. When a diabetic has heart problems, I always
find *Hawthorn Garlic Capsules* from Alfred Vogel very helpful. Of
course, it is extremely important that a good balance of a
carbohydrate-protein diet is adopted to reduce heart disease.

Many people ask me about the Dr Atkins' diet and, certainly
for diabetics, it might be of help. However, with the fatty, high-
protein foods that are allowed in that diet, other problems will
probably arise and, therefore, as humans are meant to have a
balance of proteins and carbohydrates, I find individual diets for
each person necessary, most certainly for diabetics. We see this
especially in the use of meat or high-cholesterol food products.
It is well known that game and chicken are a lot better for a
diabetic than red meat. Some researchers have been very busily
proving this. Cholesterol and protein levels can be measured in
the urine. A normal protein diet has been proven to be very
helpful for diabetics. A lot of people who have used the Dr
Atkins' diet have reported indigestion to me. Therefore, I repeat
that an individual diet is so much better. Researchers have
concluded that digestive tract symptoms with diabetic patients
can be linked to diabetic complications, especially peripheral

neuropathy, nerve damage or poor control of sugar levels. The latter is especially true with Type II diabetes. One has to change one's lifestyle and food products because of it. A sufficiency of nutrients and the right kind of food are required for efficient digestion, absorption and gastrointestinal health and comfort, with proper elimination.

The fundamental design of the human digestive system is a tube and, like all other animals, we spend our physical lives passing organic matter through this tube, processing it as it goes and extracting those nutrients we need to grow and maintain ourselves. How good we are at this can determine our energy level, longevity and state of body and mind.

Over a lifetime, no less than 100 tons of food passes along the digestive tract and 300,000 litres of digestive juices are produced by the body to break it down. Our 'inside skin', or gastrointestinal tract, is 30 feet long with a surface area the size of a small football pitch. It is constantly being renewed; in fact, most of the billions of cells that make up this barrier between us and the inside world are renewed every four days.

The gastrointestinal tract itself has high nutrient needs because of high turnover of epithelial cells and synthesis and secretion of digestive enzymes.

Some digestive enzymes are important. One I particularly like for diabetics is *Digestizyme*:

Each capsule delivers:

Lipase	100 LU
Amylase	2,100 DU
Protease	6,500 HUT
Glucoamylase	4.95 AGU
Cellulase	200 CU
Bromelain	64,000 PU
Papain	50,000 PU

The enzyme activity is measured and expressed in Food

Chemical Codex (FCC) units, the national standard for plant enzymes.

Other ingredients: sugar beet fibre, gelatine and magnesium stearate.

Usage: Enzymes are proteins that catalyse reactions with a high degree of specificity and efficiency and they are present in all living organisms. Digestive enzymes are secreted into the digestive tract to break down food matter into its component nutrients, which can be absorbed across the gut wall. If this enzyme system does not work effectively, optimal health cannot be maintained because of the failure to absorb the nutrients needed.

This product provides broad spectrum vegetable-sourced enzymes which digest protein, fat and carbohydrate. As well as by diabetics, *Digestizyme* may be used by:

- The elderly
- Those recovering from an illness
- Smokers and alcohol consumers

Dosage: One capsule at the start of each main meal, up to three daily, or as directed by a practitioner.

Contraindications, warnings: None known at the recommended usage.

Side Effects, over-usage: None known at the recommended usage.

We often see that digestive problems occur when you overindulge in certain foods, especially when alcohol drinkers become subject to diabetes. Those who drink too much alcohol have an increased risk of being diagnosed with diabetes. Again, taking everything in moderation is the right thing to do.

I once read a report in the research magazine *Health Which?*, produced by the Harvard School of Public Health in Boston, that on a Western diet one has an increased risk of developing Type II diabetes. I feel very strongly about this and, during my years of practice, I have seen the success of so many patients who were willing to stick to good dietary management. I have also seen that smoking during pregnancy can increase a child's risk of becoming diabetic later in life.

An article in the *New England Journal of Medicine* 2002; 346: 393–403 states that the risk of Type II diabetes can be reduced with lifestyle changes – this is without doubt. Research has found that lifestyle intervention can be more effective than even *metformin* (a diabetic drug) in reducing Type II diabetes, and sticking to nutritional guidelines is of the greatest importance for diabetics.

The Karolinska Institute in Stockholm has carried out lengthy studies on this, as discussed in the *British Medical Journal* 2002; 324: 26–7. With Type II diabetics, but also with other patients who are too often overweight, obesity can hold a risk factor of arterial disease or heart or circulatory disorders. The risk of developing a lot of these problems can be prevented if one controls one's own weight. In the following chapter on dietary management, I will give several pointers on how to do so. I cannot over-emphasise the fact that it has been proven that people with Type II diabetes are nearly twice as likely as those without diabetes to be diagnosed with venous blood clots: according to the *Archives of Internal Medicine* 2002; 162: 1182–9, obesity is associated with nearly three times the risk of developing such a complication.

Stress management, which can improve blood glucose control, has been the subject of studies in many universities, and reducing stress levels (as with the young man mentioned at the beginning of this chapter) is of great benefit. While I was teaching this young man some breathing and relaxation exercises, I also used colour therapy, and the colour magnetic lamps that I often use were very helpful for him. These lamps also achieve great results in diabetics with retinopathy. It has been suggested in *The Lancet* 2002; 359: 251–3 that damage to the retina, seen in people with diabetes, might be due to oxygen deprivation to the inner layers of the retina when it is dark at night. This proves again my theory on the endocrine system that you can often see, by looking at the eyes, what is going on in the body. Researchers have concluded that people with diabetes might even benefit from sleeping with night-time illumination.

Looking at all these different ways of altering your lifestyle, it is clear that diabetes management can be improved. It is necessary to establish a healthy diet, supplemented by vitamins, minerals, trace elements and some amino acids, which I very often use to treat Type II diabetes. Nature's Best produce a very good remedy called *L-arginine*; this is an amino acid known to stimulate the secretion of insulin by the pancreas.

Often one's lifestyle can become restricted due to the problems created by being diabetic, but so much can be done to help overcome this. A middle-aged lady came to consult me. She thought her life was over because of her diabetic foot ulcers, but she found great relief when I gave her some *St John's Wort* and *Horse Chestnut* (two favourite remedies of Alfred Vogel); I also used *Curapulse*. It is difficult to heal diabetic foot ulcers, but this electric stimulation treatment is very helpful (it can also be used to accelerate wound healing). After that, I gave her some acupuncture and prescribed ointments from the well-known herbalist, Abbots of Leigh in Lancashire. This combination of treatments healed the nasty ulcers that were caused by the lady's diabetes and afterwards her lifestyle changed so much that she could lead a normal life again – she was even able to attend her granddaughter's wedding.

The nutritional guidelines for American diabetics have recently eased somewhat. One of the biggest changes is that the American Diabetic Association (ADA) has relaxed its dietary restrictions on high sugar-content foods. New guidelines say that controlling a total of carbohydrates is more important than just avoiding sugary foods. This, of course, brings a responsibility, because a lot of diabetics who have read about it have relaxed too much. As I often say, the spirit is very willing, but the flesh is weak. It is so easy to give in to just the odd biscuit or cake, or a small amount of alcohol, but sugar, alcohol and nicotine are very addictive substances and therefore it is better to be strict with your diet and respect these foods as much as possible. I remember very clearly when the Canadians and Scots arrived in Holland during the German Occupation. That was the first time I had ever seen chocolate. When they came into our town in their jeeps and gave out chocolate, I went home with a little piece. My mother divided it into four and said, 'Taste this.' I told her that I had never tasted anything like it and, of course, I wanted more, but she said, 'No, you should respect this all your life.' Being careful with sugar and respecting it, as well as carbohydrates, is vital in order to maintain a healthy lifestyle. Although it seems very appealing to relax one's diet, especially when it comes to sugar, I have to disagree with the ADA – it is not the best thing to do.

It is vitally important that a healthy diet is followed and, if it is not adequate, that organically grown foods are added for extra vitamins. Vitamins, minerals and trace elements are very important in this day and age, when the immune system needs careful attention. One simple vitamin can make a very big difference. In *The Lancet* 2001; 358: 1,500–3, I read about tests where babies were given supplements of vitamin D; the results showed that the inclusion of this additional vitamin led to a lower risk of the children developing Type I insulin-dependent diabetes. The study involved 10,000 children born in 1966 in Oulu in Lapland, Northern Finland. These children were followed until 1997 and it was found that the ones who had *not* been given vitamin D supplements were considerably more likely to develop the disease, whilst those suspected of having rickets (caused by a vitamin D deficiency) during the first year of life were three times more likely to develop the disease. By making sure that babies had adequate vitamin D supplements the researchers proved that the trend of an increase in Type I diabetes amongst children, pointed out by Dr Murray, could be slowed. It is most important that a good balanced diet, supplemented by vitamins, is followed. I remember that just after the Second World War nearly every doctor or paediatrician prescribed drops of vitamins A and D which, at that time, was very important because of deficiencies caused by rationing. This went on for years.

I have mentioned the endocrine system often in this book and the importance of balancing the hormonal system, because of the influence that this has on various periods of life, such as premenstrual tension, or even during the midlife crisis in men. It is quite interesting to see that young women with Type I diabetes are known to start their periods later and are more likely to have irregular periods than women without diabetes. Some studies found that, with Type I diabetes, women with diabetes were also likely to reach the menopause at a younger age. When problems occur around these particular periods of life, it is beneficial to take some extra vitamins, minerals and trace elements to balance the hormonal system. We have clearly seen, in studies carried out by the Women's Royal Voluntary Service, that with menopausal or menstrual problems, the vitamin theory and the application of it have been very beneficial. Good results have been found with *Optivite*, a remedy from Nature's Best, which contains:

Table 10: Nutrients in Optivite

Vitamin A	375 mg (1250 IU)	Magnesium	41.6 mg
from Vitamin A Palmitate	250 mg	Zinc	4.2 mg
Beta-carotene (750 mg)	125 mg	Iodine	12.5 mg
Vitamin D	0.4 mg (16 IU)	Manganese	1.6 mg
Vitamin E	11 mg (16.6 IU)	Copper	83 mg
Vitamin C	250 mg	Chromium	16.6 mg
Thiamin (Vitamin B1)	3.4 mg	Selenium	16.6 mg
Riboflavin (Vitamin B2)	4.2 mg	Choline	52 mg
Niacin (as nicotinamide)	4.2 mg	Inositol	4.2 mg
Vitamin B6 (pyridoxine)	50 mg	PABA	4.2 mg
Folic acid	33.3 mg	Betaine HCl	16.6 mg
Vitamin B12	10.4 mg	Citrus	

Bioflavonoids	42 mg		
Biotin	0.01 mg (10 mg)	Rutin	4.2 mg
Pantothenic acid	4.2 mg		
Pancreatin	15.6 mg		
Iron	2.5 mg		

All minerals in the above formula are presented as amino acid chelates.

Other ingredients: calcium amino chelate, potassium amino complex, stearic acid, microcrystalline cellulose, hydroxy-propylmethyl cellulose; colour: titanium dioxide, magnesium stearate, silicon dioxide, magnesium silicate; and flavouring: natural mint.

Usage: *Optivite* is an excellent nutritional supplement for women of menstruating age, who are often at risk of a deficiency of certain nutrients in their diet, such as iron. *Optivite* can help correct multiple dietary nutritional deficiencies for such women and contains significant amounts of vitamin B6 (pyridoxine), other B vitamins, iron and magnesium. Six tablets per day should be taken for three menstrual cycles before results are seen.

Dosage: One to three tablets twice daily, or as directed by a practitioner.

Tea, coffee, other tannin-rich foods, e.g. red grapes or their juice, as well as alcohol may significantly interfere with the absorption of some constituents of *Optivite*. Those taking *Optivite* should be advised not to consume these to excess and to avoid them completely for one to two hours both before and after ingestion of the supplement.

Contraindications, warnings: Persons on oral anticoagulants should be monitored as vitamin E may increase the action of drugs such as warfarin.

This product contains vitamin A. It should not be taken if pregnant or likely to become pregnant, except on the advice of a doctor or antenatal clinic.

Very often, in combination with *Optivite*, I prescribe *Female Balance* and other supplements that help maintain the hormonal balance. *Female Balance* provides essential vitamins and minerals that are depleted in women who experience premenstrual syndrome (PMS). These critical nutrients are combined with concentrated extracts of herbs that women have depended on for centuries. *Female Balance* was formulated exclusively for Enzymatic Therapy by my son-in-law and myself.

Dosage: Three to six capsules daily during periods of PMS as an addition to the everyday diet.

Table 11: Nutrients per three capsules of Female Balance

Essential vitamins and minerals:

Vitamin A (beta-carotene) (non-toxic form of vitamin A)	16,665 IU
Vitamin E (D-alpha tocopherol succinate)	200 IU
Vitamin C (ascorbic acid)	200 mg
Magnesium L-Aspartate	150 mg
Pantothenic acid (D-calcium pantothenate)	100 mg
Thiamine HCL (vitamin B1)	50 mg
Riboflavin (vitamin B2)	50 mg
Calcium citrate	50 mg
Iron (ferrous succinate)	18 mg
Zinc (gluconate)	15 mg
Chromium (polynicotinate)	250 mcg
Folic acid	100 mcg
Vitamin B12 (cyanocobalamin concentrate)	50 mcg
Selenium (L-Selenomethionine)	50 mcg

Other ingredients:

Dong Quai extract (4:1) (angelica sinensis)	75 mg
Liquorice root extract (glycyrrhiza glabra)	60 mg
(standardised to contain 5 per cent glycyrrhizic acid)	
Milk thistle extract (silybum marianum)	50 mg
(standardised to contain 70 per cent silymarin calculated as silybin)	
Black cohosh extract (4:1) (cimicifuga racemosa)	30 mg

Chaste berry extract (5:1) (vitex agnus-castus)	20 mg
Pyridoxal-5-phosphate	10 mg

Contains no sugar, salt, yeast, wheat, corn, daily products, colouring, flavouring or preservatives.

It is very important that each individual looks carefully at his or her lifestyle, taking into consideration his or her symptoms, background and previous history. Each diabetic is different and reacts differently, as we saw when research was conducted into the efficacy of animal and human insulin. For nearly 60 years, people with diabetes who required insulin treatment were prescribed animal insulin – originally beef insulin, in the 1970s mainly pork, and now highly purified beef, pork or human insulin. In 1982, genetically engineered so-called human insulin received marketing approval. It was claimed for a while that human insulin would be better as it was anticipated that it would not produce antibodies. However, none of these claims and expectations proved to be founded. During the mid-1980s, there were widely circulated false rumours that animal insulin would be discontinued. Within a year of the changeover, people started to report loss of, or reduced, warning symptoms of hypoglycaemia, more severe hypos, and generally more problems in controlling their diabetes safely. Further research was undertaken and the adverse effects experienced by some people taking human insulin have had a long-lasting influence. I always feel that if diabetics are insulin-dependent, well-balanced dietary management and some extra vitamins, minerals and trace elements are necessary, as I have mentioned throughout this book. There is no evidence after 20 years' research that human insulin is of more benefit clinically and, as I have said before, it is important that each case should be looked at individually. Sometimes one comes across the greatest surprises and it is a learning process to see how each diabetic reacts.

Sustained improvements in lifestyle not only increase the quantity of life, but more importantly, the quality. Prevention is better than cure. When the initial symptoms of diabetes surface, it is crucial that these should be investigated. Even on the outside of the body, there are many signs to indicate that something might be wrong inside. I often find this with cranial osteopathy, which I have practised for many years. In balancing the endocrine system in the cranium, one can discover exactly where there are imbalances and this often indicates that something is wrong elsewhere in the body, as is the case with reflexology. These simple forms of diagnosis have saved a number of people from running into more serious conditions later on and if the indications are that either Type I or Type II diabetes is present, strict control is necessary. I am very impressed, as a diabetic, that this disease is so well managed in hospitals today. However, our health is our responsibility and to obey the rules is very important. With complementary therapies, a lot can be done to back up the treatment that is given in hospitals. I have seen too often that when patients do not obey the rules they can develop problems with their eyesight, limbs, even leading to amputation, and other serious health problems. The kidneys and adrenals play vital roles in the endocrine system. As I have said before, if one causes a problem, they all cause problems. Harmony between them all is of the utmost importance. There is basically no excuse in the world we live in today, where there are plenty of medical organisations, hospital consultants and complementary practitioners, for a diabetic not to live a normal life with all the excellent help available.

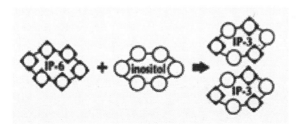

There are seven endocrine glands,
Seven colours in the solar spectrum,
Seven layers of light receptors in the eye retina,
Seven basic scale steps in the musical octave.

~ CHAPTER SIX ~

What about Dietary Management?

The other day, a little girl sat in front of me. She had an insulin-dependent diabetic condition, in addition to quite a lot of other problems, and she told me about her diet. This little girl of five, who was very conscientious and straight to the point, took her diet more seriously than many adults. She knew exactly what was right and what was wrong for her to eat and drink and adhered to all her dietician's instructions, and rightly so – her health depended on the balance of a good diet.

Many people struggle on diets and are tempted to eat the wrong foods. Sugar is often a killer to a diabetic, but so too can be the wrong dietary management. The countless patients I have seen over the years usually have no trouble in starting a diet, but they often lose interest after a while and start to think that they can eat this and that. There are so many views on diet and all the specialists who have written on the subject never seem to agree on what are the right and wrong foods. However, one thing they do all agree on is that sugar is very dangerous for diabetics. Nevertheless, I can sympathise with many patients who ask me why one book suggests one thing and another suggests something completely different. This causes huge problems with dietary management. Each expert has a different viewpoint, so it is very difficult to get them all to agree on a special diet. The reason for that is, of course, that everyone is different and every diet has to be tailored to their individual problem areas. Some people need more protein than others, and others need more carbohydrates. The secret is to find the right balance, not only in the acid-alkaline system, but even more importantly in the proteins and carbohydrates. This is probably one of the most important areas in a diabetic's diet. There are diabetics who make a remarkable recovery if they give up potatoes – not because the potato is bad but, as a carbohydrate and a nightshade vegetable, for some diabetics it can act as a poison. Others may have a lot of problems with wheat. I am therefore a great believer that there should be an individual diet for every single person.

When I learned that my blood sugar was 33, I immediately stopped eating potatoes and sugar (in any shape or form), and cut my consumption of bread right down. The improvement in my health seemed almost like a miracle when I excluded these products from my diet. Over the years, I have realised what is good for me and what is bad. Being Dutch, my favourite vegetable was the potato and I have unfortunately had to give this up altogether, because the minute I reintroduce potatoes into my diet, my blood sugar begins to rise and continues to do so. I have added a whole lot of extra vegetables into my diet, such as leeks, cress, sauerkraut and other leafy vegetables. I have cut down on cabbage as, again, I noticed that this particular vegetable brought about an imbalance in my blood sugar. In that respect, I agree a little about the blood group diet and would possibly even go as far as to agree partially with the Dr Atkins' diet. However, there is a lot of common sense in adjusting the diet for each individual. One can be one's own best doctor, and will feel that if a particular food is not agreeable, then it should be omitted from the diet. When one experiences discomfort – a bloated tummy, flatulence or irregular bowel movement – it is helpful to look at dietary management, or even go so far as to have some allergy tests carried out to discover the offender. It is of the utmost importance that the diet should be kept on the right lines.

Proteins and carbohydrates need to be very finely managed. Food combining is a very good idea, and eating proteins or carbohydrates singly is sometimes of importance. Basically, though, humans are designed to have a balance between proteins and carbohydrates. That should be one of the primary considerations, not only for a diabetic – for everyone.

I have a habit of sometimes changing my diet. One of the best diets I have tried is the one that Alfred Vogel designed for diabetics. That particular diet is very important for a lot of diabetics and I will outline it later in this chapter. However, when I am travelling, it is sometimes difficult to follow properly and I have to adjust accordingly. I know the problems diabetics often face in trying to follow a specific diet, because I travel a lot and sometimes have to eat the food provided by the airline. It is a sad situation that in hotels, restaurants and aeroplanes, food is very often inadequate or does not cater for people with dietary problems. It amazes me that in a world with so many diabetics more provision is not made by offering the right food and drink. Dietary management is an important matter and although there are many different diets, it would be very helpful if the importance of having the right foods for people on special diets were promoted.

Another important factor in the diet is eating the right foods when free radicals start to accelerate. Free radicals are natural substances in the body and, when they are under control, everything is fine. However, if there is an acceleration it needs to be controlled, otherwise this can lead to other illnesses and disease. In a diabetic's diet, it is important to eat the foods that mop up the extra free radicals that can affect the whole system. Sometimes we may not like these foods, such as broccoli, spinach and tomatoes, but other foods that mop up free radicals, such as salmon and other fish, which are very appetising. If you want to know more about this it would be a good idea to study my book, *The 10 Golden Rules for Good Health*, which gives a lot of information on dietary management.

As I have said, when I first discovered I was diabetic, I decided that I really wanted my life to continue without any controlled drugs, so I took the remedies I have talked about and went on Alfred Vogel's diet. I keep sugar, salt and simple carbohydrates (such as white bread and other refined products) low, balance proteins with carbohydrates, and feel very fortunate that I can still work 92 hours a week without too many problems.

Overall, then, good dietary management is essential for the diabetic. We are what we eat, we are what we drink, and we would all benefit greatly from taking a little extra care and looking closely at our diet. Patients often promise me they will stick to their diets but this does not always happen. Sadly, if we don't take care of our bodies, then we have to pay the price, and that can be the high price of losing our life, as I have seen so often throughout my many years in practice. It is just a question of making up one's mind and realising that it pays to invest in one's own health for the future. I cannot stress this matter enough.

I remember talking to a lady at great length about how important it was for her to give up the delicious truffles that she loved so much – and chocolate cherries, another vice. I emphasised that they were going to kill her. After much effort to try and get my message across, I told her that there were so many things she could eat instead and listed them all. She told me she really liked fruit. I spelled out what kind of fruit she could eat, but she went home and tucked into grapes, bananas and other fruits that are not advisable for diabetics. After two days, the lady came back and said she was bursting with sugar after taking my advice. I asked her to tell me what she had done. She had eaten pounds and pounds of grapes, which she thoroughly enjoyed: her blood sugar was far higher now than when she was eating chocolate cherries and truffles. Of course, I told her the reason –

fruit sugar is very quickly absorbed by the bloodstream. I had to talk to her again to try and get her to understand what foods she could eat safely. Believe it or not, when I mentioned nuts, she told me that she loved walnuts. Well, that was lucky. I told her that if she cracked open a walnut, the 'brains' – the soft tissue within the walnut shell – was worth its weight in gold for a diabetic. I advised the lady that she could add walnuts to salads or whatever she liked, but that she should not throw away the shells until she had one pound of them. Then she could put them into a pint of water, boil it for at least half an hour and drink the water – either cold or hot, whichever she preferred – and that she would see her blood sugar lowering in a few days. That was her salvation. She could not believe that by drinking little glassfuls of the walnut water each day her blood sugar had taken a turn for the better within a week. She told me that from 12, it went down to 7.4. She was so happy. Now she has given up the chocolate cherries, truffles and grapes, and has reduced the bananas and other very sweet food. The excellent results of drinking the walnut water gave her the motivation to carry on and she can now cope better with her diet. In a simple way, she said something that I have often felt. After doing her very best, she was so often disillusioned when she went to the hospital or to her doctor, only to be told that there was very little change. The reward for trying her best was so little that she did not feel it was worth the bother. This is the advantage of combining a complementary method with the treatment prescribed by your doctor, dietician or hospital: you are taking some responsibility for your own health and when you see improvements, you will know that you have done it partly by yourself.

There is a lot to learn from nature, and a lot in nature to help us. How wonderful it is to see what a simple food like bilberry can do for a diabetic, or perhaps some periwinkle added to one's salad with a dressing of *Molkosan*. There are many things that can be done to help bring down the blood sugar, then you can reap the rewards for the effort you have made.

Here is Alfred Vogel's diet for diabetics, taken from his book, *The Nature Doctor*.

A DIET FOR DIABETICS

Diabetics need to pay special attention to their diet. In contrast with most other diseases, diabetes makes one want to eat more. To solve the problem of diet, it is important to eat an adequate amount of food, with the proviso that it does not consist of too many carbohydrates. This can be achieved by eating primarily vegetables, which are rich in vitamins but low in carbohydrates. Lacto-vegetarians can obtain their protein requirements from milk products, especially sour milk, buttermilk and soft white cheese (cottage cheese or quark). If one is used to eating meat, this should be restricted to small quantities of lean, muscular cuts of meat. The following menu for one day can be taken as a model.

Breakfast

Take your pick from buttermilk, sour milk or cereal coffee (Bambu). For a change, you can sometimes have yoghurt. Make sandwiches using rye bread, flake bread, wholemeal bread or crispbread. There is also a special diet crispbread available for diabetics. Spread the bread with soft white cheese, such as fermented skimmed milk cheese or cottage cheese. Garnish the sandwich with tomato slices or culinary herbs, such as parsley, chives or freshly grated horseradish. If you prefer fruit for breakfast, follow my second menu:

Bambu coffee with cream, fruit muesli with rye flakes, whole rice flakes or All Bran. Use only fresh fruit in season. Bilberries (blueberries), blackcurrants and apples are particularly beneficial. Add some sesame seeds or grated almonds, but no sugar. When the berry season is over, use natural fruit juices with no additives.

Midday Meal (Lunch)

Soya mix rissoles, creamy cottage cheese or curds with horseradish and a seasonal vegetable, either steamed or au gratin. In addition, a large plate of salad made up of various raw vegetables is most important. Make your choice according to what is seasonally available. White cabbage, raw sauerkraut with no additives, lettuce and, above all, plenty of cress and nasturtiums, are excellent. Prepare a dressing from *Molkosan* and cream; whey is very good for activating the pancreas. For this reason, diluted *Molkosan* is also recommended as a drink. For a change, have a cup of Bambu with a little cream after your meal. What you should avoid, however, are beverages containing chemical additives.

If you like meat, another typical menu is as follows: grilled veal or beef, steamed vegetables and a mixed salad, as explained in my first example. Choose either diluted *Molkosan* or sour buttermilk to drink.

Evening Meal (Supper)

You would do well to eat only a light meal at night. For this reason, follow the suggestions given for breakfast. For a change, you might try the following: vegetable or sesame soup, a vegetable baked in the oven or steamed tomatoes, and a small plate of mixed salad or raw natural sauerkraut.

Introducing Variety

You must allow for a little variety, however, so that the diet does not become monotonous. This can be achieved by varying the combination of the items mentioned or varying their preparation. If loving hands prepare the food, it is always possible to find new ways of presenting it. For instance, diet pasta for diabetics can be used instead of soya mixes, bran mixes or sesame dishes.

Horseradish and cress have a healing effect on the pancreas and should be used as often as possible. From time to time, mix in a little finely chopped mugwort, another herb which has a beneficial effect on the pancreas. Diabetics can also use onions to season their food. Another good seasoning is yeast extract. Spread *Herbaforce* extremely thinly on bread and cover with onion slices. This is excellent for the pancreas because it includes both yeast and onion. A word of advice for diabetics is to make a conscious effort to eat slowly, chew everything well and salivate properly. This will help the body to utilise the food more effectively and will satisfy one's hunger more quickly. Even though the diabetic has a greater craving for food, it is not advisable to eat too much, since the excess will only place a greater demand on the digestive system. For this reason it is extremely important that the patient eats only natural wholefoods that are rich in nutrients.

Diabetics and those who suffer from obesity can also derive benefits from juice days. In addition, diabetics should acquire the habit of taking a glass of Alfred Vogel's mixed vegetable juice with every midday and evening meal.

As far as obesity is concerned, in diabetics it can be of the normal kind or hypophysial, although the latter is very rare. Alfred Vogel's mixed vegetable juice diet is of great benefit in the case of normal obesity. It is recommended to take nothing but juice, together with rice crispbread, for two or three days every week. At the same time, support the stimulation of the endocrine glands with a seaweed preparation, preferably on an empty stomach in the morning. Good results have been gained with *Kelp* tablets. This, incidentally, helps to combat early-morning tiredness too.

A fast day, eating only apples and grapefruit, beside the vegetable juice days, is also beneficial and helps to reduce weight. At any rate, grapefruit is well suited to reducing excess weight. For this reason always add half a grapefruit or the juice to your muesli in the morning and evening. If you are prone to obesity, make it a point to eat half a grapefruit with your breakfast every morning. Furthermore, reduce your intake of protein to 40 g (1½ oz) and also limit carbohydrate intake considerably; try to meet your daily requirements by eating wholegrain products. On the other hand, you may eat salads to your heart's content.

Molkosan can help diabetics a great deal. If you want to assist the digestion, add a teaspoon or tablespoon of *Molkosan* to a glass of mineral water and drink this at mealtimes. Of course, you do not have to take mineral water, ordinary water will do just as well. *Molkosan* regulates the secretion of gastric acid; it reduces an excess of acid and increases its quantity when there is a lack of it. It also benefits diabetics because the lactic ferments stimulate the pancreas, so it is without doubt one of the best drinks for diabetics.

Regular use of *Molkosan* will lower the blood sugar level and, at the same time, reduce the quantity of sugar in the urine. Of course, an appropriate natural diet must be observed too. A little patience is necessary, but after several weeks, a positive change for the better will be noticed.

Having an efficient pancreas is important for obese people, as this gland influences the fat metabolism. Regular use of *Molkosan* will slowly reduce excess weight, especially if kelp tablets are taken at the same time. This does not mean, however, that people who are underweight will have to avoid taking whey concentrate, for it regulates the metabolism rather than having a specific catabolic effect. So both underweight and overweight persons will benefit. In short, *Molkosan* makes for better assimilation of food.

Molkosan can also be applied externally: it has proved to be more valuable in the treatment of pimples, eczema and cradle cap than many other expensive preparations. For the most part, eczema can be treated by dabbing on undiluted whey concentrate. In cases of skin impurities and blemishes, good results are achieved if it is both taken internally and applied externally. Where athlete's foot and nail mould have not yet yielded to any other remedy, *Molkosan* will give quick and reliable relief. Just soak some absorbent cotton in it, bind this on the affected part and leave it on overnight. Dr Devrient of Berlin has confirmed that no other remedy for mycotic diseases is quicker and more reliable than *Molkosan* whey concentrate. When used to clean minor wounds, scratches and cuts, it is a first-class antiseptic. For incipient tonsillitis or during the course of this disease, painting the throat with whey concentrate is most helpful. In fact, if it is done in the early stages, it may well prevent the disease altogether, especially when *Lachesis 10x* is taken at the same time.

Many years ago, I drew attention to my experience in the treatment of internal and external carcinomas with whey concentrate. Frequently, the mere swabbing of external cancerous growths and skin cancer has proved very effective. I vividly remember one special case of a cancerous tumour on the calf of the leg. When the surgeon had removed it, he told the nurse in attendance that he felt doubtful about the wound ever healing. Still, we swabbed it with *Molkosan* and, to the surgeon's astonishment, it did heal very well and quickly. Other successful cures have been achieved by giving whey concentrate orally and externally and I am happy to say that Dr Kuhl, having made his own experiments, now acknowledges the importance of lactic acid in the treatment of cancer.

Of course, I do not wish to say that such lactic acid preparations are a panacea, a cure-all, but they have certainly brought the treatment of cancer a step further along the road. Because *Molkosan* has a fairly high percentage of natural lactic acid, it is of immense value in an anti-cancer diet. As a drink, diluted with mineral water, it is both prophylactic and curative in its effect. Dr Kuhl also recommends raw sauerkraut for this purpose, because of its lactic acid content. It is, indeed, a great pleasure to see how the experiences and observations we began to report on in our magazine and books many years ago are now being confirmed as facts.

Once you are familiar with the many benefits of whey

concentrate, you will appreciate and stop wondering why, in the past, high-ranking personages did not consider it beneath their dignity to take 'whey cures' for the benefit of their health.

Horseradish (Armoracia rusticana)

Since horseradish is one of the healthiest seasonings there is, it should be used much more in the kitchen. It is rich in vitamin C and is the best-known dietary remedy for scurvy, only raw sauerkraut being equally effective. Horseradish has a regenerative effect in cases of dysbacteria and helps to overcome functional disorders of the pancreas, such as diabetes. It is a good seasoning agent for diabetics, being curative at the same time. If you use it as a seasoning in the spring, in small amounts but regularly, it will also help in the fight against 'spring fever'. It has been discovered that horseradish contains a considerable amount of antibiotic substances, including a kind of penicillin, which explains why horseradish syrup is so effective in cases of throat diseases. Also because of its antibiotic properties, horseradish tincture is of great benefit when treating wounds that are not healing well or are forming scar tissue. Even when other remedies have proved ineffective, horseradish tincture will not only bring relief surprisingly quickly, but will actually cause the wound to heal.

For home use, tincture of horseradish may be prepared in the following manner: grate some fresh horseradish, mix it well with pure alcohol and let it stand for an hour or so. Then filter it through some gauze or muslin. The resulting tincture can be used on wounds, cuts and grazes as an antiseptic. Although it may sting somewhat, it will be most effective and the pain and soreness will quickly disappear.

Grated horseradish can be used in place of onions when these, applied as a poultice, have not succeeded in stopping, for example, a bad headache. Simply apply the grated horseradish to the back of the neck.

Horseradish, being one of the spice plants that have a reliable medicinal effect, should be grown in your garden, if you have one. It will then always be available. Add horseradish to carrot salad and the latter will be less sweet and more palatable; many men, especially, prefer it in this way. The flavour of cottage or curd cheese is also improved by horseradish, and the same is true of salad dressings.

Always mix a little grated horseradish into your salads. In addition to making the salad taste better, horseradish will reduce any tendency to colds and chills.

For older people, horseradish, as well as garlic, is a most excellent medicine. Both regenerate the blood vessels, especially the arteries, and reduce the blood pressure. If you are over the age of 40, you should give these two remedies serious consideration. They serve an important purpose, act in a regenerative way, and are stimulating.

However, you must be careful not to use too much horseradish, since it is very strong. The Chinese make a horseradish relish that, if eaten without knowing, will take you by surprise as the pungent flavour goes up your nose, indeed, it seems, even to your brain, causing temporary discomfort. The sensation is severe and definite, as with any other strong stimulation, but do not forget that the effect is also one of cleansing.

Mugwort (Artemisia vulgaris)

Apart from an essential oil and a bitter substance, this herb also contains inulin, a substance similar to a carbohydrate, but one that is tolerated by diabetics, unlike ordinary starch and carbohydrates. This makes it possible for the body to receive natural sugar-like substances without the need to engage the pancreas (the islets of Langerhans) in their digestion. Diabetics should take advantage of mugwort. The finely chopped leaves can be used in salads as an additional flavouring. In former days, mugwort was also well known as an ingredient for stuffing geese and ducks. In fact, this is still the custom in some areas.

Salt

Those who suffer from kidney ailments know that little or no salt is one of the important rules of their treatment if they are to recover rapidly. So, even for those in excellent health, it would be sensible to reduce our salt consumption as much as possible so as to avoid overburdening the kidneys. That the kidneys are healthy is especially important for diabetics, as we have seen. We should definitely give more consideration to these facts, since many other diseases and ailments also require a low-salt or salt-free diet in order to protect the kidneys or effect a cure.

HELP FOR THE PANCREAS

Papaya stimulates the pancreas and helps to digest protein. If you happen to indulge in too much protein, eat some papaya and you will find that the feeling of fullness and listlessness disappears in a matter of minutes. No wonder, then, that *Papayaforce*, which is made from papaya leaves and the juice of unripe fruit, is such a helpful natural product. In fact, *Papayaforce* has proved to be an excellent remedy for a range of pancreatic problems, including fatty stools caused by insufficiency of the pancreas, even typical pancreatitis. *Papayaforce* should preferably be taken in conjunction with *Kelpamare* because of the latter's potassium iodide content. Diabetics will benefit from *Papayaforce* too, since it is a great aid in digesting fat and protein. Anyone who suffers from diabetes should take two *Papayaforce* tablets after every meal and will be delighted at the effect of this natural remedy.

If you intend to travel to a subtropical or tropical region, even if only for a short visit or vacation, do not forget to take some *Papayaforce* with you. Remember, two tablets after every meal can save you from a lot of trouble. It is much better to pay a little attention to your body and care for your health than fall victim to amoebic dysentery or a stubborn worm infection.

URINE TEST

Having been aware of the value of a urine test, we should not consider it extravagant to have a comprehensive examination at least once a year. On several occasions, I have been able to detect diabetes through a urine test. In these cases the patients complained for years about tiredness and thirst but no one had ever linked these symptoms with diabetes. The urine analysis, however, proved it beyond a doubt.

JAN DE VRIES HEALTHY EATING PLAN

If you have a tendency to be overweight, for a few weeks it might be beneficial to follow a carefully formulated diet that Alfred Vogel and I worked out many years ago, which is as follows:

Note: the secret of success with this diet, as with all diets, is carefully weighing your food each time. All soups must be made using stock cubes and vegetables only. Cream soups may be made using part of your daily milk allowance.

Daily Allowances

Milk – half a pint fresh or semi-skimmed, or one pint skimmed, or two small cartons plain yoghurt or low-fat fruit yoghurt
Wholemeal Bread – 3 weighed ounces, *not slices*
Meat – 4 oz, or Fish – 6 oz, or Smoked Fish – 4 oz, or Chicken – 5 oz
Fruit – 3 portions

Weekly Allowances

Butter or margarine – 4 oz or 'Gold' – 8 oz
Cheese – 8 oz
Eggs (optional) – up to 7
Exchanges for 1 oz of bread
Potato – 3 oz
Crispbread or crackers or water biscuits or two plain biscuits

Breakfast cereal – 1 oz of any sort except sugar-coated
Porridge –1 oz *uncooked* weight
Cooked rice – 2 dessertspoons
Variety is the spice of life.

Meats

4 oz daily, cooked in any way except fried
Beef, corned beef, kidney, lamb, liver, mutton, tongue, tripe,
sweetbreads, veal

Fish

6 oz daily cooked in any way except fried (4 oz smoked)
Crab, cod, haddock, halibut, hake, herring, kippers, lobster, ling,
mackerel, mussels, oysters, pilchards, prawns, salmon,
sardines, shrimps, trout, tuna

OR

Poultry and Game

5 oz daily cooked in any way except fried
Chicken, turkey, rabbit, grouse, pheasant, venison

Eggs

1 medium egg daily (optional) cooked in any way except fried

Cheese

1 oz of the following except cottage cheese
Caerphilly, Camembert, Cheddar, Cheshire, Cottage (4 oz),
Danish blue, Edam, Gruyere, Leicester, Parmesan,
Roquefort, Stilton, Wensleydale, smoked Austrian

Vegetables

No restrictions – artichokes, asparagus, aubergines, bean
sprouts, Brussels sprouts, beetroot, broccoli, cabbage (any
type), cauliflower, celery, carrots, cress, cucumber, courgettes,

chicory, leeks, lettuce, marrow, mushrooms, onions, peppers, pimentos, parsnip, pickles, parsley, fresh and runner beans, radish, swede, spring onions, spinach, tomatoes

In moderation – avocado, baked beans (3–5 oz), beans (broad, butter, haricot), chickpeas, peas, sweetcorn

Fruit (three portions daily)

Apple – 1 average; apricots – 2 fresh; bananas – 1 small; blackberries – 4 oz; cooking apples – 1 large; dates – 1 oz; damsons – 10; gooseberries – 10; grapefruit – half; orange – 1 average; peach – 1 average; pear – 1 average; pineapple – 1 slice fresh; pomegranate – 1 small; plums – 2 fresh; raspberries – 5 oz; strawberries – 5 oz; sultanas – 1 oz; tangerines, etc. – 2. Unsweetened fruit juice – 4 fl oz

Drinks

Tea, Russian tea, herb tea, coffee, Bambu, Bovril, Oxo, Marmite, soda water, lemon juice, tomato juice, water, Energen 1 cal, slimline drinks, low-calorie tonic

Seasonings

Salt, pepper, vinegar, mustard, lemon juice, herbs, spices, Worcestershire sauce

Points to Note

- Your daily allowance must be consumed within a period of 24 hours.
- Eat your weekly allowance within one week.
- You may eat as often as you like within your allowance.
- You must not eat fewer than three meals a day.
- If a food does not appear on the list, do not eat it without prior consultation.

If we look at Alfred Vogel's diet or my health diet, it is clear that one has to cut out sugar totally.

In view of the demands of today's ever-increasing pace of life, it is of paramount importance to care for our body at least as much as we look after our car. We all understand that it is more economical to rectify a problem with the car when it first shows up, before a major repair job becomes necessary through sheer neglect. Does our body not deserve the same consideration? Take, for example, our kidneys and think of the great demands they are subjected to; much pain and discomfort can be avoided later if prompt attention and constant care are given to them.

~ CHAPTER SEVEN ~

What about Sleep, Exercise and Meditation?

It is undoubtedly of the greatest importance that a diabetic gets enough sleep. Insomnia is one of the worst problems for a diabetic because, during sleep, the lymphatic system is very active, and the lymph glands cleanse the waste material that the body gathers during the day. It is therefore essential to get sufficient sleep in order that the lymphatic system can do its work properly.

Our busy life today suffers from a lack of balance, with an unequal distribution of physical and mental work. We are often over-taxed and do not take enough exercise for the body which, consequently, diminishes our ability to relax. This is a really sad situation.

If insomnia is a problem, sprinkling a few drops of lavender oil on your pillowslip can be of great benefit. It is also helpful to look at your eating pattern. In the evening, while watching television, one often feels like nibbling on crackers and cheese, but these particular snacks will keep one from sleeping. A healthier alternative would be a good walk round the block. Going to bed on a full stomach – especially after consuming foods that are not conducive to sleep – will only end up causing you additional problems.

Herbal tea (for instance lemon balm tea) is the best thing to drink at night if you have sleeping problems. Taking soothing herbs can also help, for instance 25 drops of *Valerian hops* half an hour before going to bed. There are also other natural remedies and tablets for insomnia that can be useful and are not addictive or habit-forming.

The breathing exercise that I always advocate will be of help (see p.105). A warm bath with aromatherapy oil can aid relaxation – a clean body is part and parcel of a good sleep. Even taking simple measures like these may be sufficient to overcome this problem.

Poor circulation can prevent a proper sleep, but this can be helped with a hot water bottle or bed warmer if you cannot warm up naturally. Better still, take a foot bath, or alternate hot and cold baths, to warm your feet. A warm shower or bath is recommended when the body has cooled and will not warm up. If you do have poor circulation, never go to bed with cold feet because it can keep you awake for hours. In that case, it is best to have a warm bath.

Sleeping drugs are the worst thing anyone can take because they do not cure insomnia, unlike natural remedies. Those who do not subject themselves to the laws of nature as regards sleep and rest can become the slaves of chemical drugs, constantly resorting to sleeping pills. If you have been used to taking these drugs, cut them down gradually. Relaxation can do much more for you than medication.

As Alfred Vogel said, salutary sleep means learning to go to bed early. Soft harmonious music, not loud, may send you to sleep, and uplifting reading has a calming effect, in contrast to exciting television entertainment. Quietly meditating on the deeper meaning of life can free us from the sickening happenings of our times and help us find the necessary rest.

So then, salutary sleep is based on many small necessities and requirements. Give due consideration to them before you consult your doctor about insomnia, because the answer to your problem is generally to be found simply by observing them.

SLEEP, THE REMEDY WE CANNOT DO WITHOUT

The best medicines, money and possessions cannot take the place of sleep. When travelling, it may overcome us on a train or plane, to the homeless it may come as a relief in open fields, and at night it gathers the more fortunate ones among us into its soothing arms on soft pillows. It is always necessary and we should not drive it away, otherwise it may one day take revenge by avoiding us.

Do we really know what sleep means to our senses? Do we show understanding for its necessity? Have we ever stopped to think about how it recharges our batteries by letting us rest and relax? While we are asleep, we forget everything. When a day has been full of heavy burdens, we can bring it to an end by means of merciful sleep. For the nerves, brain, muscles and blood vessels it is an important break. While we sleep, millions of body cells rest and renew themselves. Sleep remains a mystery, a phenomenon of nature, in spite of all that has been written about it.

Since it is said that every cell is subject to a rhythm of tension and repose, it is astonishing to hear that millions of heart cells, from before our birth to the last moment of our life, never stop working. It is strange that not all cells have been given the same potential. While some require the regular rhythm of rest, others are capable of working throughout life with untiring pliability, without ever resting. What miracle makes this possible is known only to the One who put the building blocks of life together, and who gave them life in the first place.

AN EXTRAORDINARY THING – THE NEED FOR SLEEP

One thing we know for sure from experience: we must not let

the body go short of sleep since there is simply no substitute. Experience and observation also tell us that bedtime has to do with the coming and going of daylight. We are aware of the fact that sleep before midnight is more refreshing and relaxing than sleep afterwards. If we postpone our bedtime to the hours after midnight, we will not derive the strengthening benefits from sleep that we would by going to bed earlier, because the hours before midnight provide double the benefits. Not everyone needs the same amount of sleep. Individual requirements generally lie between six and ten hours.

If we want to derive the most from sleep as a source of energy, we must definitely make sure that we allow ourselves the time we individually need. Those who cut sleep short so that they can work more will soon realise they have calculated wrongly. During the day, energy will decline and efficiency will diminish. If we need a great deal of sleep in order to feel fresh during the day, we should not compare ourselves with those who get by with less. We must, somehow, obtain the amount we personally need. We should never forget the mysterious renewing power of sleep. It is essential for good health.

If sleep causes a problem, there are so many healthy alternatives that can be used to help this situation. Diabetics in particular need help when sleep is impossible and should do everything they can to alleviate the problem. Often when nothing else helps, I have found electro-acupuncture of great benefit. A few sessions of this particular treatment will help restore a good sleeping pattern.

It is also a very good idea to make time for exercise. That the body makes good use of oxygen is of the utmost importance for a diabetic and exercising will help with this. Walking, swimming and cycling are all enjoyable ways of exercising. Health and fitness is very important and, today, it is considered an integral part of our lives. The vascular system, the lymphatic system, the circulatory system, the digestive system, the immune system and the respiratory system are all profoundly dependent upon physical activity for their efficient functioning. On an emotional level, we benefit immensely from the reduction of stress and anxiety, lethargy and depression that exercise brings. It can also provide significant relief for those suffering from insomnia and irritability.

Different types of exercise all have their own particular benefits. The amount of oxygen generated during yoga, for example, is very important for circulation. In addition, the hormonal system also benefits. Another form of light aerobic exercise is line dancing, which is great fun. Joining a keep-fit class makes exercise enjoyable, but make sure that you join a class that is suitable for your own particular level of fitness. Your doctor can, of course, advise you on your fitness level.

CORRECT BREATHING

I read so much in the press about the terrific benefits of breathing exercises. Many years ago in China, when I worked in a hospital, I met a young doctor who was full of energy. She told me about a famous Chinese breathing exercise – also called Hara breathing – and I am grateful that I managed to take a short course in this method of correct breathing. The technique involves too many exercises to mention here, but I would like to share with you the one I do myself each day.

About four o'clock in the afternoon (that is the time I was born, and it is well known that most people get tired around the same time of day as when they were born – so if you were born during the night, you are lucky!), I lie on the floor and tell myself to relax completely. I close my eyes and tell every part of my body from head to toe to relax, until I feel as if I am sinking deeper and deeper into the floor. Then I place my left hand about half an inch beneath my navel and place my right hand over it. At that point, a magnetic ring on our vital centre – the Hara – is formed. The Chinese have an old saying that the navel is the gauge to everything that happens and certainly, by doing this exercise, I feel very relaxed. After that, I breathe in slowly through my nose, filling my mouth with air, while keeping my ribcage still. This sounds easier than it is, but it actually takes a little time to master properly. Concentrate your mind on your stomach and breathe in slowly. Once your stomach is filled with air, round the lips and slowly breathe out, pulling in the muscles to flatten your stomach. This can be done as often as desired. The sensation after finishing this exercise is normally either one of complete relaxation and a desire for sleep, or of refreshment and the desire to return to work. I must stress that you should breathe naturally, just as a baby would do. It sometimes helps to imagine walking in the garden, with a beautiful scent of flowers, and inhaling slowly to smell that perfume. Once you have taken a deep breath, you will feel the pressure when inhaling and exhaling at the back of the palate of your throat. Continue with this deep breathing by taking three more inhalations and exhalations – this will be enough for your first time. This is often of the greatest possible help and will provide the relaxation that one needs. I cannot over-emphasise the importance of breathing properly.

I wrote an article a long time ago that it is appropriate to repeat some of the content from now. It was called 'Life is Breath and Breath is Life'. This quote, from one of the ancient eastern texts, shows that throughout the ages great civilisations have paid particular attention to the breath. Our society, on the other hand, seems to overlook this simple truth. It is possible to live without other faculties such as speech, sight, hearing and healthy limbs, but without breath, life would not exist. It is the whole basis of life, the central foundation from which other bodily functions begin. For instance, the heart would cease to function if the breath did not begin the process and, being the very basis of thought and movement, it provides the energy which activates the brain and the body. It is the most essential element of life itself. Breathing not only affects our bodily functions, but our mental attitudes and our emotions as well.

We do not have to remember to breathe, for it is purely automatic. That is, the relationship between brain and body functions automatically at all times. Yet we do have a great deal of control over this vital function. We can, by conscious decision, slow down the breathing rate by decreasing it to several times less than its normal rate. During periods of mental or physical stress, the breathing becomes fast and irregular, causing undue strain on the heart and raising the blood pressure. Practice in breath relaxation will calm an irregular heart rate and hypertension may be reduced, if not alleviated. Changes in the breath pattern can be brought about relatively quickly, the state of mind can be controlled and the whole bodily functions brought into a state of ease and harmony. Only by being aware of the breath do we have the basis of helping ourselves to combat our emotional, mental or physical problems.

The nervous system depends on the breath for the bulk of its vital energy. The nervous system is concerned with the function, regulation and control of the whole body. As I have already stated, it is often unfortunately cut down or restricted due to the influence of stress, depression etc. These problems reduce the volume of breath taken in which, in turn, cuts down the amount of energy absorbed into the body, resulting in the nervous system lacking in full vitality, leaving the body in poor condition and open to infection by all sorts of bacteria. Mouth breathing also reduces our energy intake because we are bypassing the nerve energy pick-up points in the nostril tract. Children who grow up as mouth breathers usually have lowered vitality and a weakened constitution.

The importance of nostril breathing cannot be over-emphasised. The narrow passages of the nostril and respiratory tract provide an intricate and purifying system of warm mucous membranes and tiny hairs, which prevent dust and impurities from entering the lungs, to be expelled by the outgoing breath. The delicate cell structure of the lungs is protected by the warming of the breath through the nostrils. In recent years, there has been increasing medical awareness that symptoms of many different illnesses can be traced back to a disruption of the natural breathing pattern and, certainly, many of the stress-related illnesses may be brought under control or even alleviated by correct and harmonised breathing.

The essential features of respiration are the transference of oxygen from the atmosphere to the tissues and of carbon dioxide from the tissues to the outer air. However, it is very important to keep the relationship between the oxygen and carbon dioxide in balance because oxygen, whilst essential to body functioning, can also be a toxic substance unless it is absorbed and used in the correct quantities, with the right balance. Most people think of carbon dioxide as being a poisonous gas to be eliminated from the body as quickly as possible. This is only partly true, because a certain amount is necessary for the correct and delicate balance in the complete process of respiration. For example, in cases of hyperventilation, the level of carbon dioxide becomes too low, resulting in dizziness until it again reaches its correct level.

The renewal of air in the lungs is secured by the respiratory movement of inhalation and exhalation. The thorax may be thought of as a box which alters its shape and size during each respiration. On inhalation, the cavity of the thorax is enlarged and the lungs, being elastic, expand to fill up the increased space. This expansion of the lungs causes air to be sucked in through the upper air passages. On exhalation, the cavity of the thorax returns to its former size and carbon dioxide is expelled from the lungs. This increase in size of the thorax cavity is brought about by the upward and outward movement of the ribs, and the downward movement of the diaphragm. When at rest, the diaphragm is dome-shaped, having its cavity towards the abdomen. It is attached to the bottom of floating ribs at the front and to the spinal column at the back. When the muscle of the diaphragm contracts during inhalation, it becomes flattened and therefore depressed towards the abdominal cavity and this, in turn, results in movement of the ribcage.

However, if the trunk is not erect, the muscles between the ribs cannot do their work of moving the ribs, and diaphragmatic movement is therefore impaired. In fact, the more stooped the posture, the less movement can be achieved by the diaphragm and the lower the energy level becomes. This shows the need for erect posture, with the spine being upright and the chest kept open. We should try to encourage this without putting any undue stress or tension on the body.

Isn't it wonderful to think that we actually have a great deal of control over this marvellous process – the breath! We can learn to restore a natural, relaxed breathing pattern, for only if the breath is truly relaxed does the body feel at ease and, in turn, the mind becomes more calm and peaceful.

Learning to control the breath needn't be a complicated process, with lots of breathing exercises that are difficult to master. One of the simplest ways to start is by learning to observe the breath, and you will be surprised at how effective this is in bringing about the calm and relaxation you desire. This exercise may be done lying down, sitting in a chair or even standing, so long as the spine is straight and the chest open. If possible, the eyes should be closed to aid concentration and to reserve energy. Observe the breath and the movements within the chest and abdomen. In truly relaxed breathing, the movement is from the abdomen and the whole breathing process is rhythmic and smooth. The 'out' breath is the most important, it being in itself a relaxation, normalising the body, and it should be slower than the inhalation. Try to observe the slow, gentle movement of the abdomen, and allow this regular breathing pattern to help you relax which will, in turn, help you to regularise your breathing. To start with, you can even say to yourself, 'I am breathing in' and 'I am breathing out'. Remember, there should be no strain on the breath at any time, for this only causes tension within the body.

Try to practise each day and you will notice that the feeling of relaxation in the breathing will bring with it a wonderful state of mental well-being. If we practise regularly and learn to gain gentle control over our breathing pattern, we will be creating a good, firm basis for our daily lives, by being able to control the tensions and stresses that now seem an inevitable part of modern-day living.

MEDITATION

Meditation is a tremendous form of relaxation. To meditate upon the positive aspect of a problem is of the greatest help. One could say that prayer is possibly the purest form of meditation. Positive meditation and wanting to get well and have the body in complete harmony is the best way to help the endocrine system, as it is not only physically and emotionally, but also spiritually, of the greatest importance that harmony is restored. The pituitary gland, which is so strongly linked with the cosmos, will react strongly to prayer and meditation. Therefore, it is important that the whole endocrine system, which is guided spiritually, is in harmony in order to lead a fit and active life. When the body is ill, there is disharmony. In order to get better, strive to balance whichever part of the body is out of harmony. I have often seen with patients who are under a lot of stress and anxiety that prayer and meditation can help a great deal. I ask them to sit down and teach them how to meditate. A good form of meditation is as follows:

First part

Sit down in an armchair, your head resting, your feet flat on the floor. Breathe calmly and hear your breath going in and out. Now take a very deep breath in and, when expiring, say to yourself, 'Relax.' Do this three times.

Now you are going to relax all the muscles of your body. Begin with your eyes and mouth. Squeeze your face tightly together and then suddenly let go. Feel a wave of relaxation travel down your body. Consciously relax your neck, shoulders, arms, hands, tummy, back, upper legs, the calves of your legs and feet.

When you have done this, try to remember a nice spot where you like to be – a lake, a mountainous area, a holiday spot etc. Imagine you are there, and stay with that memory for a couple of minutes. This is the preparation for the exercise.

Second part

Now you are going to *see* your illness. For illustration, I shall refer to the spine, but you should visualise whichever part of the body causes you problems. You are going to *see* with your mind's eye gloomy, grey patches in your spinal cord that do not look bright. You are going to *see* with your mind's eye how the bodily defences deal with it. You can *see* blood vessels opening, bringing a flood of healthy blood loaded with vitamins. You can *see* cells building, restoring the fatty layer around the nerve track. If you want to imagine the thing as electric wires being restored with new insulation being put around them, then that is all right, as long as you *see* with your mind's eye how, with the help of vitamins, minerals and the body's own defence system, the spinal cord is restored to its function. You may use your own imagination as long as you see your illness as *weak* and your bodily defence as *strong*.

Now, when you have finished this mental picture, you are

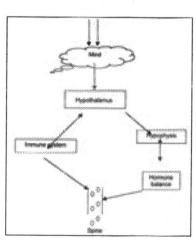

going to see yourself quite strong again. You see yourself walking normally, full of vitality. Pat yourself on the back for having done so well. Breathe deeply three times, then open your eyes.

Do this exercise three times a day: when you wake up, at lunchtime and before you go to sleep. Be in a quiet room. Never skip an exercise. Do not *force* yourself, just *see* it with your mind's eye. That is enough. What you're really doing is putting a new (and healthy) programme into the computer. It may take you six to twelve months before the new programme starts to work out in your body.

Meditation is so important. It is of great benefit to understand what goes on inside your mind and body, and learn to recognise the problems.

Meditation is also wonderful for circulation. I once knew a young doctor who it was obvious to me had bad circulation; when I told her that she called me a 'nutter' and said there was absolutely nothing wrong with her circulation. So I gave her a little leaflet which I had prepared many years before and asked her to fill it in quickly for me. I have given it below:

Are Circulation Problems Affecting Your Health?
  Answer these important questions: YES/NO

- Do your fingers and toes often feel cold?
- Do you find your arms or legs often going to sleep?
- Do you feel a numbness in your limbs?
- Do you get cramp in your hand when you write a letter?
- Do you often feel a tingling sensation in your lips or fingers?
- Does a short walk cause you aches and pains?
- Is your memory as good as it should be?
- Are you sometimes impotent or frigid?
- Do you smoke?
- Does your job or home life cause you stress?
- Do you drink coffee, tea, colas or other caffeinated beverages?

When she had completed this form, I could instantly see from her answers that she did indeed have circulatory problems, affecting her to the extent that she could not fight off illness or disease. We have to recognise the problems we have – in other words, protecting oneself from illness and disease is much simpler than trying to cure an illness or disease.

Sleep, exercise and meditation are most important. When you are ill you need to think about things logically and take positive action, which will, in turn, give positive results.

~ CHAPTER EIGHT ~

What about Libido Problems?

It is a known fact that diabetics have a tendency to lack energy and interest in sexual relationships. Because of this, some marriages where one partner is diabetic have encountered severe problems. As I have said, diabetes is a problem that is strongly linked to the endocrine system, and I will reiterate that the endocrine system works in harmony – if one gland is out of tune, they are all out of tune. It is therefore very important that natural harmony – which can so easily be disturbed – be restored as much as possible.

There are many ways that one can work towards balancing the endocrine system with good results. Sometimes, it might simply take supplementing the diet with *Gingko 2000* from Nature's Best or one of the special range of vitamins that I prescribe from Lamberts or Nature's Best. Some women's problems accompanied by loss of libido can be treated with *Gynovite* or *Optivite*. Although the problem of low libido can lead to a lot of unhappiness, there are a number of remedies available to help the situation. A loving sexual relationship is very important in the life of a diabetic as it helps balance the emotions.

It is often said that diabetics can be moody. I find that a diabetic's mood can be restored with colour therapy. The computerised electro-colour machine lamps that we use are especially beneficial. Colour therapy is a very important part of the treatment of many illnesses and diseases, but I find it particularly helpful for diabetics. Again, we come back to the endocrine system, where the seven endocrine glands are all seated around the seven *chakras*, so important for the will, understanding and initiative.

Let's look at the main endocrine glands, the pineal and pituitary glands. In the Far East the pineal gland is called the 'third eye' and it plays a tremendous role, working almost like an aerial to the cosmos. From there it receives messages to be distributed to the other six endocrine glands. The pineal and pituitary glands then send messages to the adrenals and the pancreas. The pineal gland is connected to prayer and meditation, which is the elixir of life for the pineal gland. Although as yet the medical world knows very little about it, over the years I have learned that the pineal gland plays a very important role in the body. It secretes fluids that are very important in the growth and development of the sexual organs. I often see that if I work with the pineal gland in acupuncture treatments, it is extremely influential in balancing the other glands. Any imbalance in energy is often the result of the pineal gland not working to its maximum capacity. Sometimes the pineal gland is called 'the spirit of love', because it is strongly influenced by the emotions.

The pituitary gland is said to be the key to the chemistry of the whole body, influencing both physical and spiritual growth. It secretes hormones that chemically affect the cell membranes, and the chemical reactions in the body do not work properly when the pituitary gland is in any way impaired or prevented from doing its job. This gland is situated at the nasal suture, the place where the nose meets the forehead. An imbalance in the pituitary gland can cause infertility in men and irregular menstruation in women; the severity of diabetes can also be determined by the pituitary gland. It is therefore necessary that these glands receive the nourishment they need for prayer and meditation, which we spoke about in the previous chapter.

In order to function properly the pituitary gland needs a good intake of vegetable protein, which is very important for the production of hormones and also the different enzymes in the body. This gland is often called the 'master gland' or 'conductor of the endocrine orchestra' and it releases hormones to either promote or inhibit the release of other endocrine hormones. Indirectly, it controls such basic processes as rate of growth, metabolic rate, water and electrolyte balance, kidney filtration, ovulation and lactation. It responds to hormones released by the region of the brain known as the hypothalamus, and is a physical link between the nervous and the endocrine systems.

Then there are the gonad glands – the male and female sexual endocrine glands – which are essential for the reproduction of the species. The gonads produce internal secretions that are distributed by the blood in order to stimulate and revitalise all other glands and organs in the body, and therefore they also create a certain amount of external secretion. To my thinking the gonad glands have a role to play in present-day problems such as AIDS, and I believe that in the case of AIDS patients treatment with natural remedies which influence the gonads may produce significant benefits.

The seven endocrine glands are often treated with a lack of respect, and we ought to remember that they are very sensitive from both a physical and a mental viewpoint. Let us not overlook the fact that they are very closely linked to the seven *chakras*, or the seven sources of spiritual energy – the description used in the Far East for energy centres in the body whose counterparts are present in the physical body of the glandular and nervous system.

The locations of these seven sources of spiritual energy are as follows:

Pituitary gland – the ground *chakra*

Pineal gland – the 'third eye' or the forehead *chakra*
Thyroid – the neck *chakra*
Thymus – the heart *chakra*
Adrenals – the sacral *chakra*
Gonads – the root *chakra*
Pancreas – the solar plexus *chakra*

These descriptive names for the seven *chakras* indicate the need for physical care as well as spiritual exercise, if we are to help these energy centres to awaken and activate their healing powers, which are often dormant, in order to attain full harmony between mind, body and spirit. Physical and mental exercise serves to strengthen all the vital functions and to maintain good health.

Love, strength and power are all characteristics that are needed for the balanced life of a diabetic. Therefore, it is very necessary for the endocrine system to be in harmony. The seven endocrine glands are the mirror of the seven light receptors in the eye retina and the seven colours of the rainbow that surrounds us, and these are also in tune with the seven notes in the musical scale.

If we look at colour, we can see that the psychology of colour not only affects the physical body, but also influences our moods. Many colours have strong associations with some of the emotions and feelings that we commonly experience:

Red can help to overcome negative thoughts but is also associated with anger. If we have too much around us we may feel irritable, impatient and uncomfortable.

Orange frees and releases emotions and alleviates feelings of self-pity and low self-esteem. It also stimulates and renews our interest in life and has antidepressant qualities.

Yellow is noted for its ability to aid clear thinking and the assimilation of new ideas. It also builds confidence and engenders an optimistic outlook on life. However, on the negative side, dull, muddy yellow is strongly associated with fear and cowardice.

Green is the colour we often seek when under stress or suffering from emotional trauma. It creates a feeling of calmness, relaxation and has an affinity with nature. Lime and olive green, however, have sickly connotations and yellow-green, in particular, has strong associations with jealousy and envy.

Turquoise is helpful for relieving feelings of loneliness as it heightens communication, sensitivity and creativity.

Blue is associated with a higher part of the mind. It is also soothing, calming and protective. It inspires creativity, allowing us to connect with our intuitive feminine side. However, too much dark blue can be depressing.

Indigo, violet and purple all have a deep effect on the psyche and have been used in psychiatric care to help calm and pacify patients suffering from mental/nervous disorders. These colours balance the mind and help to transform obsessions and fears.

White brings feelings of peace and comfort. It also alleviates emotional shock and despair. It can give a feeling of freedom and uncluttered openness. Beware, however, of using too much white as it can isolate and separate us from other people.

Black is associated with the feminine life force – passive and mysterious. It is comforting and protective. From a more negative point of view, it can also prevent us from growing and changing. We cloak ourselves to hide from the world.

Grey is associated with self-control, evasion and non-commitment. It signals detachment and uninvolvement and can lead inevitably to loneliness.

THE MEANING OF COLOUR
What is colour?
Colour is a form of energy that plays an important role in almost every aspect of our lives. As we know, colours can be made visible to us by refracting white light through a prism. By this method we can view the colours of the rainbow. Each of these

colours has a different wavelength and speed of vibration. The colours of the rainbow, however, form only one 'octave' of light within the electromagnetic spectrum (of which there are 60 or 70 in total). It is estimated that the human eye sees only approximately 40 per cent of colours. Beyond the visible spectrum lie many other wavelengths, some of which are familiar to us as infrared, ultraviolet, gamma rays, X-rays and radio waves. Although we cannot see these wavelengths, we can detect their energy in other ways. Most of us are familiar with the heat given off by infrared waves and those who have used a sunbed will be familiar with the effects of ultraviolet.

Having established that colour is a form of energy, we are going to look at the effect that colours have on every aspect of our lives. As living beings, our forms are made up of ever-changing vibrating colours and we respond to colour actively or passively in everything we do. These waves of light penetrate our energetic system whether we are awake, asleep, sighted or blind.

How do we sense colour?

The primary sense organs involved in discerning colours are our eyes. Light rays travel through the pupil of the eye to reach the lens. The lens then bends these rays so that they come to a focal point on the retina which covers the back of the eye. The cells of the retina contain pigments which are sensitive to light and are of two types: rods and cones. As the light hits these sensory cells, it causes a nervous impulse which travels along the optic nerve to the visual areas at the back of the brain.

This may be easier to understand if we think of the human eye as a camera, the pupil being the aperture at the front, the lens being the glass lens of the camera and the retina being the film onto which the image is recorded. The process of assimilating this information could be compared to developing the film and the resulting image of colour is our photograph!

However, sight is only one way in which we can sense colour. It is also possible to develop a colour sense through our fingertips.

Many blind people are able to differentiate colours by passing their hands over an object. Some colours feel hot while others feel cold. In Russia, sighted people have been taught how to sense and identify colours through their hands. Try this for yourself and see if you can tell the difference between warm and cool colours.

Colours – uses and effects

Colour affects our senses, not only our sense of sight but also our sense of touch.

Colour affects our physical body. It can alter blood pressure, body temperature and muscular activity. It can also affect growth, sleep patterns and our immune system.

Colour influences our moods and emotions and can affect our ability to concentrate, communicate and express ourselves.

Colour is used symbolically. Down through the ages, certain colours have acquired particular significance within societies for various reasons.

The colour of food can have a direct effect on our appetite and ultimately on our health. We can learn to identify the healing powers of differently coloured foods.

Colour itself can be used to heal. The healing effects were first recognised in the 1930s when colour therapy was first introduced.

Colour can have a significant effect in the workplace, to the extent of affecting levels of productivity.

Colour can be used to visually alter the proportions of a room.

Colour can be combined to create atmosphere, drama and a sense of style.

How does colour affect our physical body?

Red is the most physical of all colours. It is the colour of blood and has a stimulating effect on our heart and circulatory system. It raises blood pressure, stimulates the adrenal glands and builds our stamina.

Orange strengthens the immune system and has a beneficial effect on the digestive system.

Yellow stimulates the brain, making us more clear-headed, decisive and alert. It also strengthens the nervous system and creates energy in the muscles by activating motor nerves.

Green has a balancing effect and helps to regulate circulation. It brings physical equilibrium and relaxation.

Blue lowers the blood pressure by calming the autonomic nervous system. Dark blue stimulates the pituitary gland, which regulates our sleep patterns. Turquoise helps in warding off infections.

Indigo has narcotic qualities and indigo light can be used to induce anaesthesia for minor operations. It is linked to the pineal gland.

Violet suppresses hunger and balances metabolism. It also has a purifying and antiseptic effect.

Colour and food

Red food: energy and warmth.

Orange food: good appetite (stimulates the brain and immune system).

Yellow food: happiness and cheerfulness.

Green food: calmness and love (balancing acid and alkali).

Blue and indigo food: good sleep (soothing and cooling).

Purple and violet food: creativity and contentment (uplifting and inspirational).

Colour and healing

The healing powers of colour were first discovered in the 1930s in both Italy and the USA, where they were used successfully in hospitals and institutions to help emotionally disturbed patients. This was known as colour therapy. In holistic medicine, practitioners look at the body as a whole, made up of three interconnecting parts. There is the physical body, the emotional body and the spiritual body. The principle behind holistic medicine is that if an imbalance occurs in any of the three bodies, the other two will also be affected.

Colour can be used to alter emotional energy. By introducing positive vibrations into the mind, we can drive out negative patterns which will be detrimental to our overall health. Colour therapy therefore treats the cause of the illness rather than just the symptoms. It works towards creating a balance within the body that helps it to ward off disease.

Since colour directly links to the subconscious, we can use it to diagnose the root cause of a problem and treat it at a deep level. This is why colour therapy has such an impact on chronic illnesses that have no apparent cause.

Colour in the workplace
The correct environment is very important. People working in places where little thought has been given to colour schemes, ventilation and lighting are likely to become ill. Mentally stimulating colours can improve motivation, enhance health and result in greater productivity. Colour can transform the working conditions of employees from a tiring and oppressive environment to one where they feel motivated and inspired. With this in mind, think carefully about your work area and write down some suggestions for improving this environment, bearing in mind what you have learnt about the effects of colour and the various ways in which colour can affect the body, both physically and psychologically.

Points to consider/bear in mind
1. Do you have the space and amount of light you need?
2. Is your workplace comfortable for you?
3. Do you have plants that lend a healing energy to your space?
4. Does your environment have the colours you like and feel you need?
5. Is the air you breathe fresh?
6. Is your workplace hot, cold, damp or dry?

7. Do you feel tired, lethargic, unmotivated, depressed, ill or frustrated?

Colour trends and predictions

Nowadays, with all the technological advances in communication and the ability to access the same things at the same time from almost anywhere around the globe, it is becoming increasingly difficult but, at the same time, more important for people to mark themselves as individual, with their own unique identity. Rather than a predominant style or trend in colours, fashion, interiors etc., there is now almost a reversal in this. People want to make their mark by being 'different' rather than the same as everyone else. This has led to a diverse range of styles with the current trends being much more of a mixture of styles rather than any one in particular. The exotic, fantastic, spiritual and natural are all very much in favour at the moment, interspersed with personal touches to create the uniqueness that people aspire to. This has resulted in manufacturers producing more original collections and limited editions. Hand in hand with this is the appeal of handmade items and one-off pieces that no one else will have. To sum up, people are reaching out for things that tell a story – a different story – their story, and the colours and fashions of today and tomorrow will need to reflect this.

We can see that colour therapy is of tremendous benefit and often releases stress that, in so many cases, can lead to or worsen diabetes, as we well know. Stress is undoubtedly an 'in' word these days. Everyone appears to be talking about it. However, let us be realistic – life without some stress would be boring: in fact, in some circumstances, a certain amount is beneficial. It is when stress becomes excessive or prolonged that the trouble starts. Stress is common to everyone, but some of us cope better than others when things start to get out of hand. Everyone, however, is capable of learning to control stress and channel it into positive energy. Many people who experience stress do so because they have stretched themselves to the limit and some become very ill before they call a halt to their fast living. We must learn to accept life and take it a day at a time.

Stress can affect us all, from those suffering unemployment to the high-powered business executive. It is possible, however, to avoid it. In fact, it is quite amazing what a positive attitude can do. Stress can be deployed either positively or negatively. A call of distress should never be ignored because many physical problems can develop from a stressful situation. However, stress responds well to relaxation and a sensible and healthy diet, and can be eased with a variety of herbal remedies.

Too much stress is one of the reasons why diabetics can lose interest in a normal sex life. However, it is too readily accepted that diabetics get frustrated and can be selfish, and these factors can also lead to very unhappy home situations. There are wonderful remedies, such as *Manpower* and *Womanpower* from Michaels of the United States, which may be able to help. Certainly, I have a lot of patients who have obtained great benefits from these remedies, which have assisted them to overcome these particular problems.

A new star has appeared in the sky that has also given some patients tremendous help in these problems. The main ingredient of *Indolplex* is diindolylmethane (DIM), a plant-derived nutrient found in vegetables from the cruciferous family. These foods have been traditionally consumed as part of the diet but have now become the focus of intensive study since the discovery that DIM may beneficially influence the metabolism of oestrogen. The therapeutic implications for oestrogen-based diseases such as breast cancer, prostate and heart disease, and other health issues surrounding the menopause and pre-menstrual syndrome, as well as imbalances in the hormones (important for diabetics), could be enormous since DIM appears to promote the metabolism of oestrogen and restore a healthy balance to the hormones.

Every day we come into contact with xenoestrogens within our environment, from our water supply, pesticides such as DDT and even from plastic food containers. As a consequence of this bombardment, we appear to be suffering from oestrogen-dependent diseases far more frequently than ever before. *Indolplex* may help to reduce the potentially damaging effects of these excess oestrogens by promoting healthy oestrogen metabolism.

Indole-3-carbinol (I3C) is another phytochemical derived from vegetables from the cruciferous family, whose active metabolite is DIM. It is, however, rather unstable and requires activation in the stomach to be converted into DIM. In contrast, *Indolplex*, which contains active DIM, overcomes the need for active enzymes within the vegetables and chemical reactions within the stomach. Thus, *Indolplex* provides many advantages over I3C and a lower dose is required to achieve the same result.

APPLICATION
In oestrogen-driven diseases
While no one will ever question the importance of a healthy diet in the battle against diseases such as cancer and diabetes, those at a particularly high risk may do well to consider specific supplements containing concentrated plant-derived isolates known to offer protection from hormone-driven diseases.

A daily diet high in vegetables from the cruciferous family is known to offer protection from such diseases as breast cancer and prostate disease, but one would have to consume at least two pounds of raw or lightly cooked vegetables every day to significantly influence oestrogen metabolism in a way that an 'at risk' individual would gain benefit. Dietary supplements such as *Indolplex* could offer a convenient answer.

In women, fibrocystic breast disease, endometriosis, fibroids and other oestrogen-driven diseases are becoming more common. These may benefit from supplementation with *Indolplex*, which appears to aid liver detoxification, thereby breaking down excess circulating hormones and promoting hormonal balance.

The oestrogen levels found in the male system are considerably lower than those found in women, but can still have considerable effects on the healthy functioning of glandular tissues, especially the prostate gland. Just as women accumulate fat in the early menopause, men tend to lay down fatty tissue in midlife. What makes the situation worse is the fact that fat cells contain an enzyme known as aromatase which converts testosterone into oestrogen. Once this cycle starts, more fat is deposited and more aromatase accumulates, further increasing the levels of circulating oestrogen. As time progresses, the prostate gland becomes affected and accumulates oestrogen. The exact mechanism behind prostate enlargement is not understood, but studies using oestrogen-binding agents show that reducing the oestrogen levels improves night-time urination. The use of DIM by men may delay the onset of prostate enlargement and its associated symptoms.

Indolplex and HRT

HRT has some established benefits, but there is a growing concern among users regarding the adverse effects of the oestrogen component of the therapy. The main cause of concern revolves around the increased risk of breast and uterine cancers, not to mention life-threatening blood clots. A recent study has also highlighted the fact that women with a history of heart disease run an increased risk of a heart attack during the first year's use of oestrogen-based preparations. DIM may be of help in such situations, since its use increases the levels of a protective oestrogen metabolite known as 2-hydroxyoestrogen. This metabolite is also associated with a lowered incidence of breast cancer and increased antioxidant levels in the body. The concurrent use of DIM alongside HRT in those who need the additional hormone therapy may be a powerful and safe way of offsetting the potential adverse side effects experienced by those sensitive to high oestrogen levels.

Description

Each tablet contains 120 mg of *Indolplex Compound* containing modified food starch, 25 per cent diindolylmethane (DIM), di-alpha tocopherol succinate, silicon dioxide and phosphat-idylcholine. Other ingredients are: calcium carbonate, modified cellulose gum, cellulose and titanium dioxide colour. It contains no sugar, yeast, wheat, gluten, dairy products, artificial flavouring or preservatives. All colours used are from natural sources.

Recommendations

Women: one tablet daily with food. If extra support is required, take two tablets with food.

Men: one tablet twice daily with food.

Warnings

Do not use if pregnant or nursing.

Harmless changes in urine colour may occur with the use of this product.

This wonderful remedy from Enzymatic Therapy now offers a new double-strength tablet, where only one is required to be taken per day.

Diindolylmethane ensures healthy oestrogen metabolism.

What do perimenopause, pre-menstrual syndrome, enlarged prostate glands and early heart attacks have in common? Oestrogen. A new understanding of healthy oestrogen metabolism is providing a nutritional approach to these and other important conditions confronting both women and men. Fortunately, phytonutrients discovered in cruciferous vegetables offer a natural approach to resolving oestrogen imbalance. Dietary supplementation with an absorbable form of one of these phytonutrients, called diindolylmethane, helps promote healthier oestrogen metabolism. Its hormonal balancing effects have revealed these midlife problems are not due to oestrogen itself, but rather to oestrogen metabolism imbalances.

What is diindolylmethane and how can it help hormones?

Diindolylmethane is a phytonutrient (plant nutrient) found only in cruciferous vegetables. These include cabbage, broccoli, Brussels sprouts, cauliflower, kale, kohlrabi, mustard, pak choi, swede and turnip. These plants have been cultivated for thousands of years and were initially used for their medicinal benefits. The connection between diindolylmethane and hormones like oestrogen has to do with similar characteristics at the molecular level. It is not an oestrogen or a hormone but, like oestrogen, it shares the common characteristic of being poorly soluble in water. Like oestrogen, it can be metabolised only by a special class of cytochrome enzymes that reside in cell membranes in the non-water part of cells. It turns out that when it is consumed in food or in absorbable formulations, it encourages its own metabolism. This special metabolic pathway for diindolylmethane, and the enzymes involved, precisely overlaps with the pathway needed for healthy oestrogen metabolism. Stated simply, supplementing the diet with diindolylmethane specifically promotes beneficial oestrogen metabolism and helps restore a healthy hormonal balance.

What is oestrogen dominance?

Middle-aged men and women experience changes in hormone production and metabolism resulting in excess oestrogen action. There are three basic forms of this common imbalance known as oestrogen dominance.

Perimenopause: in women, slower hormone metabolism in midlife can mean higher-than-normal levels of oestrogen and a deficiency in its healthy metabolites. Faltering oestrogen metabolism often occurs in women during perimenopause (the years before menopause) and is characterised by higher monthly oestrogen levels prior to oestrogen's dramatic fall at menopause. Additionally, progesterone levels fall during perimenopause, resulting in a rising oestrogen: progesterone ratio.

Middle-aged men: rising oestrogen also becomes a problem

for men during their 50s and 60s. In overweight men, testosterone is increasingly converted into oestrogen and rising oestrogen competes with falling testosterone. This corresponds to a time during which oestrogen accumulates in the prostate gland. Oestrogen is believed to contribute to benign prostatic hypertrophy (BPH).

Acquired oestrogen imbalance: this important form of oestrogen dominance has to do with inherited problems in oestrogen metabolism and influences of diet and chemicals on beneficial metabolite production. Acquired oestrogen imbalance affects both men and women.

What benefit can diindolylmethane offer?

Supplementing our diets with diindolylmethane can shift the production of oestrogen metabolites away from dangerous 16-hydroxy in favour of beneficial 2-hydroxy metabolites. Taking it in an absorbable formulation encourages active and healthy oestrogen metabolism. Diindolylmethane supports oestrogen balance by increasing beneficial 2-hydroxy oestrogens and reducing the unwanted 16-hydroxy variety. This improves oestrogen metabolism and helps resolve all three forms of oestrogen dominance.

Why not just eat more cruciferous vegetables?

Recent reports, like one from the Fred Hutchison Cancer Center in Seattle, indicates a higher intake of cruciferous vegetables is associated with a lower risk of prostate cancer. This study indicates cruciferous vegetables are protective for hormone-sensitive cancers. However, direct measurements of upward, beneficial shifts in oestrogen metabolism indicate you would have to eat at least two pounds per day of raw or lightly cooked cruciferous vegetables to derive the same benefit as two capsules of specially formulated diindolylmethane. Benefits for cervical dysplasia, PMS, BPH and other conditions have not been seen with the use of broccoli, cabbage juice, or dried powders or extracts from vegetables. Absorbable diindolylmethane formulations overcome the need for active enzymes within the vegetable and chemical reactions in your stomach to produce diindolylmethane. For similar reasons, its absorbable formulation provides many advantages over I3C, another cruciferous phytochemical available as a supplement. I3C is an unstable precursor that requires activation in the stomach to be converted into diindolylmethane. This means I3C must be taken at a much higher dose and can undergo unpredictable and undesirable chemical reactions in your stomach and colon. Diindolylmethane, in a delivery system to assure absorption, is by far preferable to the supplemental use of I3C.

What is the preferred form of diindolylmethane, according to research?

Plain diindolylmethane is just not absorbed because of its poor solubility. When taken as a supplement in a bioavailable formulation, it is well absorbed because of a unique delivery system. In this delivery system, it is absorbed at three times the amount you might derive from two pounds of vegetables. Its use in animals has been associated with preventive benefits for breast and cervical cancer. In humans, supplementation with cruciferous phytonutrients promotes breast, uterine and cervical health. In a study of cervical dysplasia, a recent report documented the disappearance of early cervical cancer over 12 weeks in a placebo-controlled clinical trial.

Supplemental use of absorbable diindolylmethane in perimenopausal women has been observed to benefit recurrent, pre-menstrual breast pain and to ease painful menstruation. Use of the bioavailable formulation at night has helped men with prostate symptoms of nocturia, or frequent night-time urination. Its use has been associated with easier weight loss in both women and men. A number of beneficial activities are attributed to 2-hydroxy oestrogen metabolites, including support for a more active fat metabolism and activity as antioxidants.

How much diindolylmethane is recommended?

To replace the diindolylmethane from healthy amounts of cruciferous vegetables in the diet, women should take a starting dose of about 15 mg per day of actual diindolylmethane in an absorbable formulation. Men should take about 30 mg per day in the same absorbable formulation, or bioavailable formulation. These amounts can be increased three to four times on an individual basis to derive needed benefits for hormonal balance and metabolism. Based on testing in men, improved oestrogen metabolism, easier weight loss and prostate health require a higher dose of diindolylmethane than in women.

Since pure diindolylmethane must be provided in an absorption-enhancing formulation, the dose for diindolylmethane sometimes specifies the weight of the absorbable formulation, which is only one-quarter, or 25 per cent, diindolylmethane. In the book, *All About DIM*, the suggested dose of 100–200 mg per day for women and 200–400 mg per day for men refers to milligrams of such an absorbable formulation. This dose range for hormonal balance corresponds to 25–50 mg per day of actual diindolylmethane for women and 50–100 mg of actual diindolylmethane for men.

What is the excitement regarding diindolylmethane and pre-menstrual syndrome (PMS)?

PMS symptoms of irritability, aggression, tension, depression, mood swings, water retention and breast pain or swelling are frequently seen in perimenopausal women. While a reduction in PMS severity has been seen with nutritional therapy, full resolution has been elusive. These interventions have included lower-fat diets and supplementation with minerals, vitamin D and herbal extracts.

PMS symptom improvement has been noted after beginning dietary supplementation with absorbable diindolylmethane. These results suggest it is able to correct the oestrogen imbalance in PMS. Torbjorn Backstrom, MD, an eminent researcher in the field, and others, have documented that estradiol, the primary active form of oestrogen, is elevated in PMS. Backstrom also has shown that the degree of estradiol elevation correlates with symptom severity. Also encouraging is the observation that the enzyme pathways promoted by diindolylmethane help metabolise pregnenolone sulfate. Pregnenolone sulfate is a brain hormone important for memory, but which causes anxiety if levels are too high. Like oestrogen, pregnenolone sulfate is elevated in PMS. Its healthy metabolism produces beneficial, immune-stimulating metabolites and may help relieve anxiety. Absorbable diindolylmethane supplementation promotes healthier metabolism of both oestrogen and pregnenolone in PMS.

What's the best supplemental approach to PMS?

A strong nutritional approach to PMS includes bioavailable diindolylmethane, chaste berry extract, vitamin D, calcium and magnesium. Synergistic interaction of these ingredients benefits PMS in accordance with its physiologic origins. An example of this synergy is the ability of beneficial 2-hydroxy oestrogens to increase progesterone production, potentiating this effect by chaste berry extract. This new nutritional approach to PMS helps with mineral and hormonal balance. Diindolylmethane works in conjunction with chaste berry extract to resolve the dominance of oestrogen over progesterone.

How can helping oestrogen metabolism benefit men?

Everyone knows oestrogen is an important hormone for reproduction in women. What is not often appreciated is that oestrogen levels, though lower than those in women, are also essential in men. However, midlife changes in men result in excess oestrogen production beyond its minimal essential level.

Like perimenopausal women, men experience a tendency to gain weight in midlife. Rising oestrogen production can result, since fat cells contain the aromatase enzyme that converts testosterone into oestrogen. Unmetabolised oestrogen creates a vicious cycle resulting in further oestrogen production. This occurs because fat is one source of more active aromatase enzymes, causing further oestrogen production and continuing weight gain. An open label study of diindolylmethane in overweight men and women showed it promoted more efficient weight loss and more active fat metabolism. In this regard, diindolylmethane is similar to green tea extract and spices like cayenne pepper. Diindolylmethane may have a role in helping to intervene with excess oestrogen production associated with obesity and male ageing.

Besides weight gain, another aspect of early ageing in men is prostate gland enlargement. It has been clearly established that oestrogen accumulates in ageing prostate glands at the same time enlargement occurs. This process is linked to difficulty with urination and frequent urination at night. The role of oestrogen is still being established in this process, but research using oestrogen-binding substances shows lowering oestrogen levels improves the symptoms of night-time urination. Use of absorbable diindolylmethane by men with the same symptoms has proven beneficial.

Can diindolylmethane help improve the safety of hormone replacement therapy (HRT)?

Despite a growing list of benefits attributed to oestrogen, which include younger-looking skin, stronger bones, more comfortable sex and better memory, women often view its potential side effects as unacceptable. Study of postmenopausal women receiving long-term HRT with oestrogen and oestrogen-progesterone combinations has revealed an unequivocal increase in breast cancer risk. Added concerns relate to the increase in the incidence of uterine cancer and increased risk of life-threatening blood clots, especially after bone fracture. Most recently, the nationwide HERS study reported the worrying finding that women with a history of heart disease had an increased risk of heart attack in the first year after starting to take extra oestrogen.

Many of oestrogen's risks can be related to a lack of its beneficial metabolites. It is now known that a lower risk of future breast cancer is associated with higher 2-hydroxy oestrogen levels. Supplementation with bioavailable diindolylmethane increases protective 2-hydroxy oestrogen and therefore may reduce the risk of HRT-related cancer. Reduction in the risk of abnormal blood clot formation related to HRT oestrogen would benefit women who suffer fractures while on HRT but also may benefit women with early heart disease. It has been known since the Framingham Study in Massachusetts that men with the highest estradiol level had the highest risk of early heart attack. Diindolylmethane may help normalise the cardiac risk in both men and women related to unhealthy or underactive oestrogen metabolism. Also, the beneficial 2-hydroxy metabolites have been shown to be powerful antioxidants, which may contribute to protecting against the early signs of atherosclerosis and subsequent heart attacks.

Conclusion

Diindolylmethane supplementation is a nutritional approach to achieving a safer and healthier oestrogen metabolism. Many of the benefits traditionally ascribed to oestrogen (protection from heart disease, healthy skin, bones and brain) may actually reside with its beneficial metabolites, the 2-hydroxy oestrogens. Diindolylmethane supplementation is a natural promoter of this specific pathway of healthy oestrogen metabolism.

We often see that women suffering with the symptoms of PMS and menopause will be greatly helped by the remedy *Femtrol*, which is a supplement that has been formulated to help women with these symptoms.

Clinical application

Vitamin C plays a major role in the health of the immune system. It is essential for the growth and repair of tissues in all parts of the body and needed for the formation of collagen. It is also needed by the adrenal glands to synthesise hormones, and the normally high levels of ascorbic acid in these glands are especially depleted during times of physical and mental stress.

Dong Quai extract (Angelica sinensis) is primarily used in herbal formulas as a 'female tonic' to treat muscle cramps and pain associated with different menstrual periods.

Hesperidin is a flavonoid (responsible for deep colours of berries, also found in skins of citrus and other fruits, vegetables, nuts, seeds, grains, legumes, tea, coffee and wine) which can be used to prevent or treat a wide variety of conditions. This particular flavonoid has been used for conditions such as bruising and circulatory disorders, including varicose veins.

Liquorice (Glycyrrhiza glabra) is soothing to inflamed mucous membranes and has a stimulating action on adrenal glands, which may help fatigue. It also has a balancing effect on hormones, helping to prevent PMS symptoms.

Chaste Berry extract (Vitex agnus-castus) has for centuries been reputed as a hormone balancer. It has been used to treat fibroid tumours and other female complaints. A rich source of phytoestrogens, which are valuable plant compounds that exert oestrogen effects, and so can also be used for menopausal symptoms.

Black Cohosh extract (Cimicifuga racemosa) can be used to relieve menstrual cramps and depression and also helps menopausal symptoms such as hot flushes and vaginal atrophy.

False Unicorn root (Helonias opulus) has proven oestrogenic activity and a long historical use in treating various female complaints.

Fennel Seed extract (Foeniculum vulgare) is particularly high in phytoestrogen and possesses a confirmed oestrogenic action.

Table 12: Nutrients in Femtrol

Two capsules contain:

Vitamin C (ascorbic acid)	100 mg

Dong Quai extract (angelica sinensis)	250 mg
Hesperidin Complex standardised to contain 50 per cent bioflavonoids	200 mg
Liquorice Root extract (glycyrrhizic acid) standardised to contain 5 per cent glycyrrhizic acid	50 mg
Chaste Tree Berry extract (vitex agnus-castus) standardised to contain 0.5 per cent agnuside	50 mg
Black Cohosh extract (cimicifuga racemosa)	50 mg
False Unicorn Root extract (helonias opulus)	50 mg
Fennel Seed extract (foeniculum vulgare)	25 mg

Recommendations

One or two capsules three times daily as an addition to the everyday diet.

Warnings

None known at suggested dosage.

The remedy *Female Balance* is also an excellent supplement, formulated by my son-in-law and me, and has been as great a success in the USA as in Britain. Many patients have asked me if they should take Viagra. I always tell patients to firstly try gingko, ginseng or Siberian ginseng, or *Manpower* or *Womanpower*.

Male diabetics could try *Masculex*, which is suitable for all ages, and is a comprehensive supplement specifically formulated to support male glandular function and to promote male vitality and well-being.

Clinical application

Vitamin E is an important antioxidant that prevents the oxidation of cholesterol and prevents initial damage to the artery, which can ultimately lead to the process of atherosclerosis. Atherosclerosis of the penile artery is the primary cause of impotence in nearly half the men over 50 who have erectile dysfunction. Vitamin E is also important in circulatory disorders and in the normalisation of hormone balance. *Wheatgerm oil* is an excellent source of vitamin E.

Liquid liver fractions may improve liver function, assist fat digestion, promote tissue regeneration and protect the liver from damage. Due to the vital role the liver plays in metabolism, *liquid liver fractions* appear to promote high energy levels due to their positive effect on metabolism. Indeed, they appear to be a remarkable 'tonic' for well-being.

Damiana Berry extract has been hailed as an aphrodisiac and is often helpful for men with impotence and other sexual disorders. It is especially effective when combined with *Gingko Leaf extract* which increases the blood circulation to the capillaries.

Saw Palmetto Berry extract has been found to significantly improve the signs and symptoms of benign prostatic hyperplasia (BPH) in numerous clinical studies. BPH describes the non-malignant enlargement of the prostate, which can pinch off the flow of urine through the urethra, leading to symptoms of increased urinary frequency, night-time awakening to empty the bladder and reduced force of urination. Saw Palmetto can improve the hormonal metabolism within the prostate gland. As a result of its multitude of effects, excellent results have been produced in numerous clinical studies, with all major symptoms of BPH being improved.

Beta-sitosterol may benefit men with BPH. One double-blind study of 100 men showed that *beta-sitosterol*, taken as 20 mg of *beta-sitosterol* three times daily for six months, improved urine flow, reduced prostate size and led to subjective feelings of improvement compared to the placebo group.

Cola Nut extract acts as a general stimulant, increasing general vitality.

Panax Ginseng Root extract enhances the ability to cope with both physical and mental stress, which can have numerous effects on the body, including disturbed sleep patterns, blood sugar imbalance, adrenal fatigue and reduced thyroid function. Additionally, erectile dysfunction often occurs when under stress and ginseng is claimed to be a 'sexual rejuvenator'. Some studies have suggested that ginseng increases testosterone levels whilst decreasing prostate weight. This indicates that ginseng may have favourable effects in the treatment of benign prostatic enlargement.

Table 13: Nutrients in Masculex

Amount per two soft-gels

Vitamin E (as D-alpha tocopherols)	100 IU
Muira Puama (ptychopetalum olacoides) Root extract	250 mg
Liquid Liver fractions (pre-digested soluble concentrate)	250 mg
Wheat Germ oil	100 mg
Beta-sitosterol	100 mg
Damiana (turnera diffusa) Leaf extract	100 mg
Saw Palmetto (serenoa repens) Berry extract standardised to contain 85–95 per cent fatty acids, 0.2–0.4 per cent total sterols, and 0.1–0.3 per cent beta-sitosterol	40 mg
Cola (cola nitida) Nut extract contains 4.8mg caffeine	40 mg
Korean Ginseng (panax ginseng) Root extract standardised to contain a minimum of 7 per cent ginsenosides	40 mg
Gingko (gingko biloba) Leaf extract standardised to contain 24 per cent gingkoflavonglycosides, 6 per cent terpene lactones and 2 per cent bilobalide	20 mg

Other ingredients: soybean oil, gelatin, glycerine, beeswax and lecithin

Contains no sugar, salt, yeast, corn, dairy products, artificial flavouring or preservatives.

Recommendations

Take as recommended by your health practitioner. In general, two soft-gels, three times daily with meals.

Warnings

If you are taking warfarin, check with your doctor before using this supplement.

It is very important to pay particular attention to energy, vitality and libido so that you can live life as normally as possible, even though you are lumbered with diabetes.

~ CHAPTER NINE ~

What is Hypoglycaemia?

One weekend, quite a number of years ago, I went to a seminar on hypoglycaemia organised by my great friends, Keith Lamont and Martin Budd. At that time, I wasn't a diabetic, but because I'd had so much contact with diabetics, I wanted to know what hypoglycaemia really was. I knew that Martin Budd had studied the topic quite thoroughly and that the seminar would be worthwhile.

In years gone by, when so little was known about hypoglycaemia and all people knew of it was that diabetics sometimes had 'hypos', one heard all kinds of different explanations as to what it was. Due perhaps to the twentieth-century epidemic of hypoglycaemia, more information about the condition has recently come to the fore. We have learned the value of a high-protein diet and the importance of being careful with our consumption of carbohydrates in order to maintain the correct balance of blood sugar.

What is hypoglycaemia? I learned at Martin's seminar that it can include symptoms like allergies, headaches, nightmares, blurred vision, depression, irritability, asthma, stomach cramps, forgetfulness, weight gain, phobias, vertigo and joint pains . . . the list goes on and on. All these could be linked to hypoglycaemia. It was at the same seminar that I learned how to conquer the condition. Since then, I have also realised how common the problem of hypoglaecemia really is, when so many people today eat far too much sugar.

Why do those with high blood sugar (or hyperglycaemia, diabetes) and low blood sugar (hypoglycaemia) have to follow similar diets? Sugar can affect people in every way – from memory to personality etc. Often people are not clear about how to avoid sugar and think it will cause no harm to take some forms – like honey, molasses etc. We often see that the relationship between sugar and fat can cause real functional problems and the questions that have arisen on this topic can be really quite intriguing. In his book on hypoglycaemia, Martin Budd has gone over several points and although sometimes the explanations can be confusing, the conclusion is not as difficult as it would seem. It is very important to know that hypoglycaemia means literally low (hypo) blood sugar (glycaemia), or an abnormally low level of glucose. Glucose is, of course, necessary as a body-builder, except when problems arise on metabolising sugar. When digestibility or absorption is a problem, it needs very careful balancing. Glucose can therefore be a 'body-builder', but if there is an imbalance it can also be a 'body-breaker'.

It is often said that hypoglycaemic people and diabetics can be difficult. This could be due to the fact that both conditions affect the nervous system. The nervous system is fed by glucose and this needs careful balancing, otherwise there will be a reduction in specific substances within the brain, which are needed for normal nervous activity. The whole system is built on the right output. As I have said, every gland in the endocrine system needs to be in harmony and it is necessary for that system to function fully so that the right messages are sent to the right places. The thyroid gland, which we have discussed, is also in close contact with the adrenal and pituitary glands, and the thyroid secretions are essential for insulin and for blood sugar balance. The adrenal glands will produce cortisone and adrenalin, which need the stimulation of the other glands to provide the link between hypoglycaemia and diseases. The pituitary gland, which is one of the conductors of these fluids and influences the adrenal glands and the thyroid, is necessary. The pineal gland has a big role to play in the emotions.

When a hypoglycaemic patient is out of balance, a lot of problems can occur, not only between couples, but also at work, where colleagues may be unsympathetic to the problems associated with the condition. The lowering of blood glucose or a reduction of glucose to the nervous system can indeed lead to some serious problems and very often makes it difficult to reach the right diagnosis. A lot of discoveries have been made about this and it is quite interesting to investigate the causes of hypoglycaemia, which can be problematic for the diabetic, but more research still needs to be carried out.

As I have said before, sometimes carbohydrates are better omitted from the diet, but certain carbohydrates are also necessary for feeding the nervous system. It is interesting to see that the breakdown of carbohydrate consumption – starch (bread, cereals, biscuits, etc.) is 50 per cent of the breakdown, sugar (sucrose) is 35 per cent, lactose (milk) is 7 per cent, and glucose and fructose (in fruit and vegetables) is only 8 per cent.

When Prof. John Yudkin, an expert in diabetes and obesity, lectured in Holland he made very significant research statements and explained the confusion over sugar. In one of the lectures I attended, he said something that I totally agree with: that sugar can be more addictive than alcohol or nicotine. I have proved this to be the case with the hundreds of people who have consulted me regarding this real problem. I have often seen the problems which have arisen because a patient has become addicted to sugar. My book, *Realistic Weight Control*, gives several examples. The many harmful effects on diabetics and hypoglycaemic patients who have this unbelievable craving have done more damage than one would ever think and I have witnessed many problems caused by the addiction. Not only do health problems arise – which can be either physical, mental or emotional – but also its addictive effect has made many people dreadfully unhappy.

It is also very interesting to see that, during pregnancy, some of these problems disappear. This again shows the close relationship between diabetes, hypoglaecemia and the hormonal system when, during pregnancy, the output of hormones take such a different route. As I have already said, hypoglycaemia is a problem that has only come to the fore in the last 50 years, whilst diabetes was recognised 3,500 years ago. In order to understand these two diseases, a lot more reading and research is required.

Whilst the normal blood sugar fasting level is about 70–100 mg per 100cc of blood, the normal level of blood sugar during a working day is about 120–140 mg. The breakdown in food passes to the liver and enables the small amount of insulin that remains after the excess glucose is converted to glycogen to pass through the body, assisting the utilisation of blood glucose. When a situation arises where the blood glucose exceeds 165 mg per 100cc, the excess spills over into the urine. That overflow level can be seen as a real problem for the kidneys and can often damage kidneys to the extent that the light receptors of the eyes can be damaged. It is interesting to see this process being followed by an experienced iridologist.

A lot of conditions regarding the hypoglycaemic patient will depend on the kind of food balance being followed. If, for instance, the patient is suffering from cholesterol problems, more difficulties can arise if these problems are not addressed. In my own case, where I have a tendency to ketosis, I often see an improvement when I am following a very low cholesterol diet.

So what advice can be given to a hypoglycaemic patient? It would be wonderful if there were a diet available that would really help every individual patient who has hypoglycaemia. Unfortunately, there is no such thing. One has to be careful with standard diets, as they do not take account of any health problems that the individual person may have. One thing is for sure, however – the daily consumption of carbohydrates must be greatly reduced. It is much more beneficial to have six small meals than three big meals a day, and to chew the food very thoroughly, as saliva contains a lot of necessary digestive material. Fat and protein intake should be spread evenly over the day and the amount of calories should not exceed 2,000–2,500 daily. One should have a very substantial breakfast and should also be very careful to avoid coffee, tea, alcohol and nicotine.

There are several remedies that can help with the problems of hypoglycaemia. One that I have worked with for a number of years here, as well as in the USA and other countries, is called *Hypo-Ade*. This is a wonderful remedy that deals with the symptoms of hypoglycaemia. Its clinical application is a dietary supplement formulated to support proper carbohydrate metabolism.

Table 14: Nutrients in Hypo-Ade

Amount per two tablets:

Vitamin A (fish liver oil)	5000 IU
Vitamin C (ascorbic acid)	200 mg
Vitamin B1 (thiamine HC1)	25 mg
Vitamin B2 (riboflavin)	25 mg
Niacin/Niacinamide	115 mg
Vitamin B6 (pyridoxine HC1)	25 mg
Vitamin B12 (cyanocobalamin)	25 mcg
Pantothenic Acid (calcium D-pantothenate)	100 mcg
Zinc (oxide)	10 mg
Manganese (gluconate)	10 mg
Chromium (polynicotinate)	267 mcg
Sodium	10 mg
Potassium chloride	100 mg
Inositol	200 mg
Pancreas extract	150 mg

Choline bitartrate	100 mg
L-methionine	100 mg
Green beet (beta vulgaris) root powder	100 mg
Adrenal extract	65 mg
Betaine HC1	50 mg
Wild yam (dioscorea villosa) root	50 mg
Pituitary extract	40 mg
Barberry (berberis vulgaris) bark of root	30 mg

Other ingredients include: cellulose, stearic acid, cellulose gum, silicon dioxide, magnesium stearate, vanillin, dandelion (taraxacum officinale) leaf, goldenseal (hydrastis canadensis) whole plant and water-soluble cellulose film coating.

The tablets contain no sugar, yeast, wheat, gluten, corn, soy, dairy products, artificial colouring, artificial flavouring or preservatives.

The recommended dose is two tablets taken three times daily with or after food.

~ CHAPTER TEN ~

That's What to do with Diabetes!

Some time ago, a father and mother came to consult me, along with their only daughter, aged about 16. They lived in a lovely rural area and were an exceptionally nice family, but I noticed that they were very upset and the parents asked if they could tell me about a traumatic experience that had recently happened to their daughter. She was a very quiet, nice girl, but I could see that something was terribly wrong and took time to listen to their story. The girl was very happy at school and had good results. She had done extremely well in one of her exams and for the first time in her life had asked her father and mother if she could go out with her girlfriends one evening to celebrate her success.

The friends went out and had a wonderful evening, until a man of about 36 or 37 asked if the girl, whose birthday it was, would go with him so that he could take her home. She went with him quite happily, not realising what she was getting involved in. Unfortunately, he took her back to his house, where he raped her and afterwards took her home, completely distraught. Her parents realised immediately that something very serious had happened. After questioning her, she finally told them the following day about the horrendous experience. The parents took her to hospital immediately, where she was given all the necessary tests. Because of this unfortunate situation, it was discovered from a blood test that she was diabetic. She might have been diabetic before this traumatic event, or the shock might have triggered the problem, but in any case, not only was the girl disturbed mentally, she felt ashamed and did not feel physically well either. The only blessing in disguise in this story was that her diabetes was diagnosed early.

I had a long chat with her and her parents, and I think that she became more comfortable talking to me when she discovered that I was a father of four daughters, and realised that I understood the situation and wanted to help her. I felt so sorry about the trauma she had endured, but tried to encourage her to think positively in tackling her diabetic problem. She asked me if I thought the awful incident was the cause of the diabetes, but I felt it was better to tell her that it had probably been lingering in her body beforehand and that it was, in a way, a blessing that it was diagnosed early. Because she was an intelligent girl, she understood that and she started to act positively towards her diabetes. When I told her that I was a diabetic myself, there was a small glimmer of hope in her eyes as she realised I could help her.

It took some time for her to get over the shock of the rape, but gradually she began to focus on the diabetes, which was luckily Type II, and started to control it. In fact, she quickly began to feel much better, especially when I put her on *Doctor's Choice for Diabetics*.

I also prescribed *Molkosan*, which helped her to lose some excess weight. It also has wonderful antiseptic properties and she started to feel much better physically as it assisted in cleansing her body of the awful trauma she had endured. She stuck to the diet religiously and often said, 'I am going to beat this because I want to get better.' As I have often said, diabetes is not an easy problem, but it is a problem that one can live with and it is possible to lead a totally normal life.

I was once consulted by a young man who was completely

obsessed with his diabetes, which is not the right attitude to have. He looked at the clock every minute; because his doctor had told him he should eat every three hours, he did exactly that. He was so obsessed that he couldn't concentrate on anything else except his illness because he felt he would die if he didn't follow his doctor's advice to the letter. That is not how to tackle the disease. When one has a problem, one has not only to deal with that problem, but must also be realistic and have a positive attitude towards life. It would be very sad if diabetes ruled one's life. Positive action is what is required.

A female patient told me recently that she felt her hormonal system had almost 'gone to pot'. I said that her hormones would be more balanced if she thought positively and took action to stabilise her hormonal system, which can be done in the ways I have discussed in previous chapters. A positive attitude always wins over a negative and it was of the utmost importance that she realised this. She said she also felt extremely nervous. A marvellous remedy that I often use for such a condition is the extract of oats, *Avena sativa*. This is a simple treatment, but it is of tremendous help to the nervous system when one is upset and anxious about a situation. It is for that reason I usually advise diabetics to eat porridge for breakfast. This particular lady's blood sugar was quite unstable and fluctuated wildly. I advised her also to take a little glass of extract of walnut shells every day. This liquid is often beneficial in helping to balance the blood sugar. She managed to control her blood sugar readings – again, nature had been of great assistance. Often I wonder about the tissue contained in the walnut – I call it the 'brain' tissue of the walnut – and its possibilities. We must not forget that it is often the small things that are overlooked that help. We saw this with the great discovery by Prof. Shamsuddin of the little ingredient called *inositol*, found in the inner wall of a minute rice grain. It is amazing to see how wonderful nature can be.

This was reinforced when an assistant bank manager consulted me. He was a nice young man, but very frustrated. He had many problems, not only at home, but also with his boss. He had great capabilities, but never got the chance to use them because he was so difficult. I talked to him at length. His sugar was very imbalanced and emotionally he was too involved in his work. I felt he was probably striving too hard for a higher position which, as I mentioned to him, often happens when one least expects it. Surprisingly, he benefited greatly by taking nothing other than flower essences. There are a whole range of flower essences which have no side effects at all – these are very gentle remedies which, nevertheless, treat situations effectively. When I initially saw him, he was very upset about something that had taken place, and so I gave him *Emergency Essence* – a combination of flowers that often give instant relief. After a little while, I gave him *Mood Essence*, but nothing else. He was on insulin, but even his dependence on that had reduced while taking these simple flower essences. When he subsequently complained a bit about tiredness, I also prescribed *Vitality Essence* and *Concentration Essence*. All these remedies were of great benefit to him. I then treated him further in order to balance his hormone system. He had problems in that direction too and I discussed that with him. Through this simple yet effective treatment, he became a different person. Luckily – although he never expected it – he was promoted to bank manager and is now doing extremely well, due to the little bit of guidance I gave him.

One often has to make up one's mind and say, 'Let's get on with it', or 'That's what I am going to do with my diabetes when I really have problems'. Diabetes is such an unpredictable condition. When one develops diabetes, each type and personality is very different. Nevertheless, it is important to deal with the disease in the correct manner.

A middle-aged lady came to see me a short time ago. She told me that her diabetes and blood sugar level was under control but, nevertheless, she was tired and had no appetite. She added that she often had spells of absent-mindedness, had problems with cramp and also with her vision. I enquired as to how often she saw her doctor or diabetic specialist. She said she felt she didn't need to see them but, as these problems were getting worse, she thought that she would come to see me. During our consultation, I could clearly smell acetone on her breath. I told her to go to her diabetic consultant immediately and to tell him exactly what she had just told me. I could see she was in a very progressive condition and that it was imperative to get her stabilised. I advised her about her diet, as she was also constipated and that problem is certainly not good for the pancreas. The consultant hospitalised her, which was certainly needed, but he was very happy with the advice I had given her about her dietary regime.

Another business official, who was diabetic and under tremendous pressure and stress, came to see me some time ago. I advised him to try my Chinese breathing exercise. I also suggested that he should meditate and, as he was very keen on swimming, to try a few methods developed by Kneipp. One of the things Kneipp did when he got out of bed in the morning, if it wasn't too cold, was to walk barefoot on the dewy grass to improve the circulation. My patient became so keen on this that he practised it almost every day and gradually felt that his blood circulation was improving tremendously. Light, sun and fresh air were also very important to him. He practised my breathing exercise, as described in one of the previous chapters, and told me that his skin had greatly improved, he was very grateful for these simple treatments that had helped him so much. Being very diet conscious, he asked for my views on carbohydrates and proteins. I advised him that good carbohydrates were necessary for the nervous system but, in saying that, he had to choose these carefully and it would also be beneficial if he ate organic foods. I suggested including organic grains (such as rye, wheat, millet, rice, oats and maize) in his diet, but restricting his intake of potatoes and bread. I told him that, for a diabetic, the fruit that is allowed and any raw vegetables should actually be consumed at the start of every meal, because this has proved to be a better combination for the digestive system. I also advised him that raw fruit and vegetable juices would be extremely beneficial to him. He was very happy with that advice. He also mentioned that he liked herbal teas, and a wonderful herbal tea for diabetics is the Dutch herbal tea, which is quite tasty and of great benefit. The combination of nettle tea and bilberry leaf tea is of great assistance in controlling blood sugar levels.

This man told me that he was advised in his youth to carry out fasting and asked what I thought about that. I believe that long-term fasting must only be carried out under the supervision of a doctor or dietician. He liked to fast for at least one day each month, but always felt awful, although much better the following day. Fasting carried out carefully is very wise, but he wasn't doing it the proper way. Although he was a diabetic, carrying out a full fasting day should cause no problem. In the morning for breakfast, I suggested that he took some fruit juice and a little natural yoghurt; at lunchtime, he could take some more yoghurt and some fruit or vegetable juice and, in the evening, fruit juice or vegetable juice. These combined calories would roughly amount to 600 and would be sufficient not to upset the normal dietary management. Indeed, he agreed that it would be much better for him to carry out this method. It is quite interesting that in Holland during the Second World War diabetes decreased quickly: I am convinced that a lot of diabetic problems can be helped with good dietary management and that it is always advisable not to overeat. The pancreas, the heart, the arteries, the kidneys and the liver all rely on healthy food. Therefore, fruit and vegetables are often much better for the alkaline system than many other forms of carbohydrate, which can lead to increased acidity. For the diabetic, it is important to keep acid levels low, and those burning up carbohydrates quickly would also benefit from a raw food diet. This is especially good for the enzyme system. Digestive or pancreatic enzymes are necessary for diabetics. It is my opinion that following a raw food diet for a short while is an extremely worthwhile exercise. It is also essential that the emotions of a diabetic are dealt with. If possible, diabetics should have as balanced a lifestyle as possible and make it their aim to deal with the illness in the correct manner.

Looking after the immune system is crucial: constipation or any infection will affect it. Hydrotherapy and water treatments are very important for the skin, the lungs and the eyes. Exercise (such as aerobics, yoga, line dancing etc) is of the greatest importance for anyone with diabetes, particularly when these are carried out in the open air – such as walking and cycling. Lifestyle has a lot to answer for. Nature wants everything to be in harmony in the body, mind and soul. A dynamic equilibrium should exist between the different hormones – which are, as I have said before, so much like an orchestra, led by both the pituitary and the pineal glands, and are very reliant on positive energy. Plenty of rest and relaxation is crucial in balancing these glands. Toxic stress is often created by excessive daily pressures, coupled with the wrong dietary management. It is necessary to have everything in balance.

Communication is extremely important for diabetics. Many think they have some sort of infectious disease and shut themselves away from the outside world. This is a very short-sighted and narrow-minded attitude, and the poor diabetic ends up living almost like a hermit. There is no need for this to happen, for with the correct care diabetics can live quite normally and happily. If there are problems in the body, one can deal with them. A healthier lifestyle is quite easily attainable, and recognising the problems that might occur is of tremendous assistance.

Getting a diabetic's hormone system into harmony is also essential. Whatever method one uses, it is crucial that hormone-related problems, which play such a major role in diabetes, are treated properly. It might be beneficial to take *evening primrose* (three tablets last thing at night) or a complex of *flaxseed oil*.

These contain essential fatty acids, which help to bring the omegas in the system into balance and thus balance the hormonal system. Taking extra calcium, iron, potassium and chromium also helps with this, and is sometimes necessary for controlling the blood sugar. I often give overweight diabetics chromium and zinc and they frequently say that their cravings for food lessen as a result. It sometimes requires only a small adjustment to make a difference.

We shouldn't make excuses by saying 'I cannot do it'. It is very often the case that when people say this, they are actually saying 'I *will* not do it' or 'I can't be bothered'. It is essential to do what one can in order to improve one's health and return to complete fitness.

I come from Holland, where everyone is obsessed with cycling. I am too, because I know, being a diabetic, how good I feel when I go along the seafront on my bicycle. Not only is it a great form of exercise; to inhale fresh air – oxygen – is necessary for the body. It is wonderful when I see how much fitter some very overweight diabetics become once I have converted them to take up cycling. One teacher I know, who used to go absolutely everywhere by car, now always cycles. Not only did he lose a lot of weight, but he is so much fitter and no longer feels constantly exhausted during the day.

I can well understand why people become frustrated because of their stressful lifestyles. Changing to a healthy lifestyle is worthwhile and an investment in one's long-term health. When we have a good lifestyle our body will be much more in tune with nature and will help us get the best out of life. We are the conductors of our own hormonal system and when this little orchestra of the seven endocrine glands, where the pineal and the pituitary glands are the main players, are in tune, a good tone will come into our lives. The five senses also play an important part in regulating the functions of our body. Influenced by the endocrine system, they stimulate the body to secrete noradrenaline, adrenaline and cortisol, neurotransmitter hormones that are essential in treating rheumatism and arthritis and keeping our nervous system under control. Very often, I notice problems occurring when neurotransmitters like serotonin are blocked; immediately the train goes off the rails. Don't forget that the train will only get to its destination if every plug is in the right socket in the signal box.

It often amazes me what the body is capable of. Positive will always win over negative and a negative thought will produce a negative action. A positive thought will overrule a negative action. It is essential that we are realistic about our lifestyle and, as diabetics, do the best we can to help our body with all the methods that are available to ensure that we attain better health.

When writing this last chapter, I was sitting in a plane. It was a misty, rainy, bleak day, and I was actually quite happy to leave the weather behind me. Not long after we had taken off, there was beautiful sunshine and, during the flight, the captain suggested that the passengers look out of the windows to view one of the most beautiful rainbows I have ever seen. It was majestic and awesome, and most of the passengers remarked on its beauty. As with every illness and disease, when things are difficult for diabetics and everything seems bleak, there is always hope on the horizon. A rainbow of good health prospects can help make us feel better. We should never think that we are a lost cause. Always be positive and take positive action in order to achieve what you want. Never give up. Things may appear bleak and often sad when we are confronted with difficult situations, but always try to focus your mind on replacing some of those negative thoughts with positive thoughts, so that you can fill yourself with joy and be grateful for each day that you are alive.

My grandmother, a very old and wise woman, who was also a diabetic, often said, 'You get out of life what you put into it.' If we try to forget about our own problems and do what we can to help others, we can receive so much in return. It is up to every individual to make their own decisions, yet how much easier it is to go through life with a positive attitude rather than a negative. If we are positive, our life has more chance of turning out for the better.

When things are difficult, I often think of my grandmother, who said, 'Let it go and leave it alone and look positively to the future.' I feel that this is such good advice when patients regularly come to me with a long list of complaints. When this happens, the first thing I ask myself is, 'How can I get rid of this whole list of complaints?' It so often takes just one positive thought to change all the problems that a patient may have. The decision to change has to be made and it needs the complete cooperation and understanding of the patient to carry the change through.

Illness and disease often become part of our everyday life, and we become so wrapped up in our own problems that we seem to forget about all the good things that have happened. I remember at one stage in my life when, within a six-month period, six of my very best friends died. I became depressed and questioned the meaning of life. However, I also thought of all the babies being born every day, and it reminded me that life goes on and that there was nothing I could do but accept the inevitable. I also thought about the friends I had lost and how each, in their own way, had played a great part in my life. Some, with the encouraging words they spoke when they were still with us, are reminders of the lives they led and their achievements, and have left us with wonderful memories. Visualisation techniques, together with a positive attitude, often help to change a thought pattern when negative thinking has become entrenched.

My old schoolmaster often said, 'You have to be a scout, a discoverer of yourself, to find out the change that is needed in order to do better.' Creating something new is extremely exciting because it is a challenge and, if we fail, then we try again. By challenging ourselves, we can determine what we are capable of achieving. This is why meditation is such a tremendous help because, through meditation, we also learn relaxation and positive mind exercises that assist in overcoming the limitations that we often feel we have.

We see this all too often in our relationships. Sometimes we don't get on with our colleagues at work or, even worse, we don't get on with our partners, but harmony is very important. Fulfilment in life is a treasure. In order to reach that, we have to examine the possibilities. Although it might be wet and bleak or foggy, we have to remember that above the clouds there is sunshine and a rainbow full of promise. If we look for it, we will find it. In nature, everything is in harmony and if we love nature, we will love others and ourselves. We learn throughout life that nature gives to us freely every day and that we too can share that love, which keeps life interesting and rewarding.

Another saying of my dear grandmother was, 'If you feel miserable and down and unwell, look around and you will always find somebody who is worse than you.' Let us remember the little sentence mentioned previously in this book: 'There are seven endocrine glands, there are seven colours in the solar spectrum, there are seven layers of light receptors in the eye retina and there are seven basic scale steps in a musical octave.' There are also seven colours in the rainbow. Wouldn't it be wonderful to find the right tune and harmony between mind, body and soul, and to achieve and conquer each illness and disease to the very best of our ability?

Index